# A Pathway to Health

# A Pathway to Health

· · · · · · · · · · · · · · · · · · · · · · · · · · · · ·

## How Visceral Manipulation Can Help You

**Alison Harvey**

*Foreword by* Jean-Pierre Barral, DO, MRO(F), RPT, developer of Visceral Manipulation

North Atlantic Books
Berkeley, California

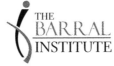

West Palm Beach, Florida

Published by              and          The Barral Institute
North Atlantic Books                   8380 Woodsmuir Drive
Berkeley, California                   West Palm Beach, Florida 33412

Cover photo courtesy of the Barral Institute
Book design by Jan Camp

Printed in the United States of America

*A Pathway to Health: How Visceral Manipulation Can Help You* is sponsored and published by the Society for the Study of Native Arts and Sciences (dba North Atlantic Books), an educational nonprofit based in Berkeley, California, that collaborates with partners to develop cross-cultural perspectives, nurture holistic views of art, science, the humanities, and healing, and seed personal and global transformation by publishing work on the relationship of body, spirit, and nature.

---

North Atlantic Books' publications are available through most bookstores. For further information, visit our website at www.northatlanticbooks.com or call 800-733-3000.

---

Library of Congress Cataloging-in-Publication Data

Harvey, Alison, 1977–
  A pathway to health: how visceral manipulation can help you / Alison Harvey.
    p.; cm.
  Includes bibliographical references and index.
  Summary: "An in-depth overview of visceral manipulation, a widely-used hands-on therapy developed by Jean-Pierre Barral to resolve structural imbalances and tensions restricting normal motion of the body"—Provided by publisher.
  ISBN 978-1-55643-901-8
  1. Osteopathic medicine. 2. Viscera—Massage. 3. Manipulation (Therapeutics) I. Title.
  [DNLM: 1. Manipulation, Osteopathic—methods—Popular Works. 2. Viscera—physiopathology—Popular Works. WB 940 H341p 2010]
  RZ342.H37 2010
  615.5'33—dc22                                                2009046156

5  6  7  8  9  KPC  21  20  19  18

Printed on recycled paper

# Dedication

To Anna Massingham, Liz Shepard, Marion Jennings, Islay, Mary Harvey, Morna Rutherford, and Gail Wetzler.

A group of strong females who have supported me on my journey in various ways. Without them, their care, love, knowledge, and their belief in me I would not be where I am today nor writing this book. I thank you all.

DISCLAIMER: The following information is intended for general information purposes only. Individuals should always see their health care provider before administering any suggestions made in this book. Any application of the material set forth in the following pages is at the reader's discretion and is his or her sole responsibility. The information and opinions presented in this book are based on the research, training, and professional experience of the author. However, the field is constantly evolving with new research becoming available, so this may alter the information presented in this book. The author, editors, and publisher are not responsible for any consequences resulting from the use of information in this text.

# Acknowledgments

My sincere thanks go to all of you, without whom this book would not have been possible:

Jean-Pierre Barral, Alain Croibier, Gail Wetzler, John Matthew Upledger, Ronnie and Nancy Allan, August Axelsson, Alex Bairstow, Hayley Cameron, Alan Garfagnini, Angus Hamilton, Rachel and Lachlan Houston, Pierre Maegaard Knudsen, Jan Ove Kristensen, Linda Linardos, Chrystal Lucas, Alice and Eleanor McLauglan, Steve and Elaine McQuade, Amy McQuater, Bob Myers, Susana Montoya-Pelaez, Tracy Naddell, Peter Legaard Nielsen, Mark O'Gorman, Christoph Sommer, Ginger Snyder, and Ann Turner. I also wish to acknowledge the work of all the teachers of the Barral Institute and thank them all for their contributions to Visceral Manipulation. In addition I wish to recognize the extraordinary effort from Dawn Langnes, Annabel Mackenzie, and Scott Russell, who have all contributed a large amount of their time and effort to support this project. And thanks to all the team at North Atlantic Books who have helped transform my text and pictures into the book you have in your hands today.

And last but not least, thank you to all my patients, who teach me more about Visceral Manipulation on a daily basis.

# Contents

# Illustrations

# Foreword

I was pleased when I heard that Alison Harvey wanted to write a book about Visceral Manipulation for the general public. There are so many people who are suffering and can be helped but may not know about this approach. I first met Alison when she was a postgraduate chiropractor studying Visceral Manipulation, later interacting with her when she served as a teaching assistant at our seminars, and then again when she sponsored our courses in the United Kingdom. Throughout this book Alison has done an excellent job of explaining what Visceral Manipulation is and how it can help you move toward greater health.

In the early 1970s in France I studied the effects of lung disease and dysfunction on the motions of the lungs. I studied patients during surgery and found that the movements and the pressure on the lungs changed with different diseases and dysfunctions. These changes also altered the motion of the supporting structures, including the bones and muscles. These changes affected the digestive system, the heart, and the neck. In fact, I observed and felt how the entire body was affected due to diseases, dysfunction, or injuries. This showed how visceral (organ) changes can significantly affect other parts of the body, and over time lead to muscular or skeletal changes as well as various symptoms, such as pain. I applied this understanding during treatment with my patients. I have treated thousands of patients, and the development of any technique such as Visceral Manipulation has always been prompted because people were in distress. I studied anatomy and then organized what to do with my hands to release restrictions. I am a practitioner first, and secondly a teacher. Students in our courses trust me because they feel that I teach what I really do in my office to help my patients.

Visceral Manipulation evaluation and treatment are done with the hands. No one argues with the wine taster who, by using his or her palate, can tell us the characteristics of a wine—its region, its vineyard, or even its vintage. The sense of touch can go at least as far. To be effective we must feel for tightness and restrictions in the body. Visceral Manipulation is not about forcing a correction on the body. It gently releases restrictions, and then lets the body take over in order to self-correct, realign, and restore health. Visceral Manipulation is about treating the patient as a whole, not just treating the symptoms.

This book is important for those seeking greater health for themselves and their loved ones. Visceral Manipulation is useful for all age groups, from tiny babies to the elderly. Do everything you can to stay healthy. Pay attention to your diet, exercise, spend time relaxing in nature, provide service, and learn how your emotions affect your health. Then if you need assistance with your healthcare, seek out a practitioner who understands the role of Visceral Manipulation in maintaining good health and helping when poor health is present.

I commend this book to all who want to learn more about maintaining their health, and I applaud Alison on her continuing dedication and contribution to the field of Visceral Manipulation.

Jean-Pierre Barral, DO, MRO(F), RPT

Grenoble, France 2010

# About Jean-Pierre Barral

Jean-Pierre-Barral is a registered physical therapist and diplomate of osteopathy who maintains a private practice in Grenoble, France. He serves as director (and faculty) of the Department of Osteopathic Manipulation at the University of Paris School of Medicine, and as chairman of the Department of Visceral Manipulation on the faculty of Medicine Osteopathy in Grenoble. He is a member of the Registre des Ostéopathes de France. He also holds a diploma from the faculty of Medicine of Paris North, one of only four osteopaths in the world to hold such a diploma. In addition, he is the academic director of the International College of Osteopathy in St. Etienne, France.

Barral began developing the modality of Visceral Manipulation in the early 1970s. In collaboration with Alain Croibier, DO, Barral has also developed the modalities of Nerve Manipulation and Manual Articular Approach based on their ongoing research. Barral is the author of numerous textbooks for healthcare practitioners on Visceral Manipulation and Neural Manipulation. He has also authored a book for the general public, titled *Understanding the Messages of Your Body: How to Interpret Physical and Emotional Signals to Achieve Optimal Health.*

# Introduction

This book has come about as part of a personal journey that has taken me from being a sick teenager to a busy practitioner running a busy multidisciplinary natural healthcare center, teaching CranioSacral therapy internationally for the Upledger Institute, and running the United Kingdom (UK) branch of the Barral Institute to provide training in Visceral Manipulation across Scotland, England, Northern Ireland, and Wales.

At the age of thirteen I became ill with Myalgic Encephalomyelitis (ME), following a severe infection from Coxsackie-B (a virus that causes flu-like symptoms) from which I just did not recover. I was one of the lucky people, if you can class anyone with ME as lucky, in that I was diagnosed within months. Myalgic Encephalomyelitis was poorly understood, misperceived, and its treatment patchy. As a result, after I had been very ill for two years and the conventional medical profession had pretty much tried out all their ideas on me with little benefit, I was introduced to complementary therapy.

Unable to go to school much, I was disabled with problems walking and writing, due to muscle pain and dysfunction, and I required several hours of sleep to recover from an hour of schoolwork. My parents took me to meet Anna, an osteopath who used Applied Kinesiology and cranial work alongside her osteopathic training. She had a new approach for me, which was to help remove dysfunctions in my body to allow my body to heal itself and thereby allow me to become well again. Through removing the physical restrictions, correcting chemical imbalances, and helping me straighten out my thought patterns to believe I could be well again, my life was totally transformed. Eighteen months after starting treatment I was able to return to school full-time to do a year and meet the qualifications to allow me to begin my career path toward complementary therapy.

By the time I was eighteen, I was well enough to leave home and travel 500 miles to train at the only internationally recognized chiropractic college in Europe at that time. While I was well enough, I still had some aftereffects and suffered a battery of infections every winter that my recovering immune system would have to battle through. Over the years, I continued to work toward health through complementary therapies, and my health continued to improve.

A decade after the onset of my illness, I thought I was well. However, I still had painful and long menstrual cycles, a sluggish bowel habit, and often felt a bit tired, but thought it was all normal. Through my interest in various complementary therapies my professional journey had led me to train in Visceral Manipulation (VM). So, deciding to practice what I preached, I travelled to receive Visceral Manipulation treatment. This was not an easy decision, but a highly valuable one for me. At the time, there was nobody in Scotland who had enough training to fully address my problems, so I sought treatment with practitioners in Amsterdam and California. After five sessions my periods shortened from thirteen days to five and became more regular and significantly less painful. With more treatment my bowel habit noticeably improved, and I had more energy and became happier in myself. Thanks to VM, I also had the excess energy that I channelled into writing this book!

I became more and more interested in VM and continued to train through the Barral Institute. Feeling that the availability and understanding of VM was very limited for practitioners and the general public in my area, I wanted to give something back to help support this work. Through this desire I became the sponsor for classes in the UK and also started to write a pamphlet on what VM is and how it works. That pamphlet grew and grew, until it eventually became the book you are about to read.

My intention is to introduce VM to you. The scope of the book is not to teach you how to practice VM, but to give you an understanding of how Visceral Manipulation can help you and why. Most of all I hope that you truly enjoy this book, and that it will help you better understand your own body and therefore allow you to be better equipped to remain healthy and enjoy your life.

The first seven and last two chapters provide general information about VM. Chapters eight through sixteen cover each organ system in our body, giving an overview of how VM helps, as well as related function and anatomy. Also included are case stories of real patients and how VM has assisted them. It has been impossible to completely remove all technical language. If you are unclear about any of the terms used, there is a glossary at the back of the book that will fill you in.

I invite you to discover Visceral Manipulation and how it may assist you and your loved ones on a pathway to health.

# What Is Visceral Manipulation?

This was the question that initially led to me write this book. It is not easy to answer, or at least not by compressing Visceral Manipulation into a few sentences, due to its breadth. And really, answering the question is the function of this whole book. However, here is my attempt to offer a summary:

Visceral Manipulation (VM) is a hands-on therapy with the specific goal of encouraging normal tone and movements both within and between the internal organs, their connective tissues, and other structures of the body where normal motion has been impaired. Additionally, other factors affecting the body may be addressed, such as tensions in the fascia (connective tissue), nerves, and blood vessels, as well as emotional issues. The ultimate goal of VM is to allow the body to self-correct, leading to improved health and optimal body function.

Visceral Manipulation is based on the premise that movement is essential for life and any restriction will affect our health. In this book the word restriction is used to mean any decrease in motion. Everything moves in space and time, and humans are no exception to this rule. This same principle applies to every structure in our bodies, including our organs. For an organ to be healthy and have optimal function there needs to be motion. Movement is transmitted between the organs and other structures of the body through a thin layer of connective tissue, called fascia. Just as when you put on a sock with a twist in it and you feel a twisting pull go up your leg, fascial restrictions may transmit a restriction in one place to other areas of the body. When you are healthy, and the fascia is flexible and unrestricted, all the structures move with a smooth, interconnected fluidity. This movement is important, as it influences activities throughout the body, from the tiniest cellular pulsations to heartbeats, breathing, and nervous system functioning. Optimum health relies upon the harmonious motion relationship among structures of the body.

Inflammation causes loss of motion of the tissues. Many factors can cause tissue inflammation, including infections, direct trauma, repetitious movement, diet, environmental toxins, poor posture, and emotional stress. As tissues heal, an adhesion or scar is formed, which is an area that dries out the fibers of the tissues so they end up arranging themselves in a different pattern than they had prior to the incident. In this way, the injury is "recorded" in the tissues and may continue to affect the body for years to come. Often it is only years later that the effects of an old injury become apparent, if they ever do. However, the altered area of tissue may be subtly impacting the movement of the area around it and creating secondary changes in function or symptoms that often do not resolve unless the original injury is addressed. For this reason VM does not focus solely on the site of pain or dysfunction, but evaluates the entire body to find the source of the tension.

Two different types of motion are important for normal functioning and are addressed by VM. The first is *Mobility,* which is the push and pull of the surrounding tissues, and how the organ is able to move and accommodate these stresses. For example, when you bend to the side, it is the Mobility of your organs that enables them to move out of the way so they are not compressed. The second type of motion is the organ's own intrinsic active motion, known as *Motility.* This is a rhythmic motion to allow fluids to move through the organ, to allow nutrients to be carried into your tissues, and to move waste products away from your tissues. Motility can be affected by a restriction of the organ or tissues surrounding it. Visceral Manipulation includes techniques to evaluate and treat areas of restriction that are affecting either a tissue's Mobility or its Motility and to thereby restore normal motion to the area concerned.

## Why Is It Called Visceral Manipulation?

The word "visceral" means the soft internal organs of the body. According to *Wiktionary*, the online dictionary, the word "manipulation" means "to handle and move a body part, either as an examination or for a therapeutic purpose." Gail Wetzler, director of the Visceral Manipulation Curriculum for the Barral Institute, came up with the phrase "organ-specific fascial mobilization," which she uses when describing VM for other medical practitioners who are unfamiliar with the techniques. This reflects the fact that VM very much works with the fascia that surrounds and supports the organs. (This will be discussed in more detail later in this book.) Additionally, it addresses common misperceptions of the word manipulation. For many, "manipulation" may conjure up images of a type of osteopathic or chiropractic thrusting manipulation. Visceral Manipulation is very gentle but still precise, without the high-speed impulses being put into the joints as is done with the thrusting spinal manipulative therapies. For this reason the word "mobilization" may more accurately reflect the gentle, soft nature of this hands-on therapy. When defined in the above terms, VM accurately describes the therapy as it was at the time of its initial development.

Jean-Pierre Barral continues to develop Visceral Manipulation evaluation and treatment techniques. He has expanded the visceral connection to pain and dysfunction to work with the joints, vascular system (blood vessels), and the nervous system. Depending on the personal interests, specializations, and direction your practitioner has followed in training, he or she may or may not have a background in all the areas now developed by Barral.

## Goals of Visceral Manipulation

*The purpose of Visceral Manipulation is to recreate, harmonize, and increase proprioceptive communication in the body to enhance its internal mechanism for better health.*
—Jean-Pierre Barral

Visceral Manipulation aims to find and resolve tensions in tissues and thereby restore normal motion to them. Jean-Pierre Barral, the developer of Visceral Manipulation, believes that practitioners of VM should "let the organism find the answer for itself." A large part of VM involves precisely identifying the structure that is causing the greatest problem for the body at that time. When teaching, he regularly says, "only the tissues know," and "let the body speak"—showing a great respect for the body's internal balance and following its lead. Throughout each session, whether during evaluation or treatment, your practitioner will be continuously feeling where the tensions are in your body and how they are responding to treatment to find your precise pathway to health. It is not possible to guess how your body is restricted, and VM depends on the principle of feeling and following your tissues to allow them to release.

While VM started with the focus of restoring normal motion to organs, it has now developed to include working with the circulatory and nervous systems. Reducing inflammation and pain by returning circulation to the body at all levels—from blood circulation in the arteries and veins to lymphatic flow at the tissue and cellular level—is a goal of VM treatment. By improving the nerve supply and balance of the body, and allowing improved functioning of the organs and sphincters (valves in the tissues) it allows the body to function more optimally. Proper muscle tone is returned by reducing the compression on muscles, which allows them to function better. Ultimately, VM aims to reestablish the body's ability to adapt and restore itself to health.

In summary, VM aims:

1. To return physiologic motion to the tissues, thereby enhancing normal movement of the body. This includes the movement of the structures in relationship to each other, as well as the motion within each structure.

2. To release and/or resolve a restriction of the tissue, including adhesions or scars.

3. To increase the rate of tissue repair.

4. To return normal circulation to the body.

5. To restore normal nerve function and stimulate nerve flow in the area being treated.

6. To increase communication within the body through improved functioning of the nervous system, circulation, lymphatic, and breathing systems.

7. To improve breakdown and removal of waste products.

8. To reduce inflammation and pain.

9. To improve the delivery of hormones and chemicals to cells.

10. To aid mood and sleep. This is partly through the effect that serotonin levels have on these issues and the role that the digestive system plays in making this hormone.

11. To normalize tone in muscles and promote normal functioning.

12. To reduce spasms or areas of increased tissue tension.

13. To return normal function to sphincters. (See Chapter Eight, "Digestive System," for a description of sphincters.)

14. To promote normal cell-fluid motion and balance.

15. To increase joint flexibility.

16. To reestablish the body's ability to adapt and restore itself to health, balance, and vitality.

## How Is Visceral Manipulation Performed?

Visceral Manipulation is a gentle therapy that locates and alleviates the abnormal points of tension throughout the whole body. It is based on the specific placement of soft manual forces to encourage the normal tone and movement of the organs, nerves, and blood vessels and their surrounding tissues. Trained practitioners use the rhythmic motions of the visceral system to evaluate how abnormal forces interplay, overlap, and affect the normal body forces at work. The treatment is through gentle compression, mobilization, and elongation of the tissues. During a VM treatment your practitioner may make a deep contact with the body, but it will not be invasive and is rarely painful, although at times it may feel as if your practitioner's hands are reaching parts others may not have reached before! These gentle manipulations can potentially improve the functioning of individual organs, the systems the organs function within, and the structural integrity of the entire body. Most patients tell me they enjoy the treatment. They appreciate feeling that I am really reaching points that seem significant to them, and enjoying the relief they experience as the tension is gently released from their bodies.

Due to the delicate and often highly reactive nature of the visceral tissues, gentle force precisely directed gives the greatest results. As with other methods of manipulation that affect the body deeply, Visceral Manipulation works only to assist the forces already at work. Because of that, trained therapists can be sure of benefiting the body rather than adding further injury or disorganization. As the source of a problem is released, symptoms will start to decrease and the body will be returned to greater health. So while your VM practitioner will not be focusing solely on treating symptoms, the changes you experience, either during a session or over the weeks that follow, are a good indication of the progression of your body's underlying state of health.

## How Effective Is Visceral Manipulation?

Over the past thirty years VM has been the life work of Jean-Pierre Barral. He has worked with tens of thousands of patients and carried out numerous research projects to validate the effects of VM. All techniques developed by Barral have proven their reliability through the work of many practitioners and have been used with hundreds of patients before being taught to practitioners who are training in VM. This means that there is clinical evidence for the effectiveness of each technique. The issue with the evaluation of VM techniques is the fact that every patient is unique. It may appear that a number of people have the same condition; however, it is likely that most of these conditions will have different causes, due to the various compensations patients have made for disparate previous incidents in their lives. The role of your VM practitioner is to find the best pathway to help your body. For this reason, for anyone to evaluate the effectiveness of VM for a particular condition is practically impossible unless it is understood that each patient may be treated with different techniques from the VM repertoire.

The final chapter of this book focuses on research that has been carried out up to 2009. In addition, throughout this book are many case reports of treatments with patients and the benefits achieved through VM.

Visceral Manipulation is an ever-growing evaluation and treatment modality, which will continue to develop as more is understood about the functioning of the human body.

### *Energy Levels Returned to Local Dad*

Gordon was a middle-aged man who was persuaded to come to see me by one of the members of his team at a local whisky distillery, where he works as the customs and excise trader. He complained of being exhausted and waking up tired each day, despite no change in his daily routine. He said he had always been a hearty eater, but recently he noticed he seemed to feel full all the time, even when he had not eaten for a while.

On feeling his body, I found the main area of restriction was around his gallbladder. I identified this through the Visceral Manipulation evaluative techniques of General Listening, Local Listening, and Inhibition, which will be described in Chapter Five in detail.

With Gordon in a seated position, I started by releasing the tissues around his gallbladder and the underside of his liver. The gallbladder is situated against the underside of the liver, and so freedom of this area is important for its proper function. Then I released the duct (pipe), which links the gallbladder into the digestive system, by helping it elongate and softening the ligaments that surround it. Finally I treated the duodenum, which is the upper part of the small intestine into which the duct flows. At this point is a valve known as the sphincter of Oddi, and this had to be balanced so that it could return to normal function. After treatment, reevaluation showed no dysfunction of this area of Gordon's body.

At the second treatment session, three weeks later, Gordon reported with delight that he felt much better and was now able to eat more normally. With this and the reduction in his fatigue he felt he had much more energy and was now able to play soccer again with his sons in the park.

2

# How Did Visceral
# Manipulation Develop?

Methods such as Visceral Manipulation have been part of the medicinal cultures in Europe and Asia since prerecorded times. Indeed, manual manipulation of the internal organs has long been a component of some therapeutic systems in Japan and China. So it's no surprise that the work of practitioners in many parts of the world incorporates treatments designed to work with the internal organs and their functions.

The developer of VM, French osteopath and physiotherapist Jean-Pierre Barral, first became interested in the idea of organ manipulation following a particular patient's case. In a YouTube video interview filmed in 2008, he describes how a man came to him with low back pain; three weeks later the patient returned and reported that his symptoms had greatly improved. Barral reports that he "felt very proud," until the patient said, "No, it's not because of you," and explained that he had seen a bonesetter who had done something to his stomach that had improved his back pain.

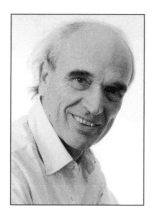

Figure 2.1. Jean-Pierre Barral

Being the curious type, Barral decided to investigate how doing something to the stomach could assist with back pain. At that time he was working in a hospital doing lots of dissections. He started looking for the connections between the stomach and the spine. He found that if he moved the stomach, it followed an axis that was the same each time; he concluded that this patterning was not just happening by chance. He also found that through various attachments and nerve and blood vessel supplies, the pattern influenced the spine. Initially he studied corpses and later worked with patients, finding the same results in both cases. One day, Barral reports, he was standing with his hand resting on an organ of a patient and noticed that although the patient was not moving, the organ was. From this he realized that every organ has an intrinsic movement that is very specific and defined, and began to study these motions. This motion he identified is known as Motility, and it allows practitioners to evaluate whether an organ is in a state of equilibrium or not.

Barral was working in the Lung Disease Hospital, in Grenoble, France, under Georges Arnaud, MD, a recognized specialist in lung diseases and a master of cadaver dissection. Working with Dr. Arnaud, Barral followed patterns of stress in the tissues of cadavers and studied biomechanics in living subjects. Often he worked with bodies of previous patients and was able to correlate what he was seeing in their tissues after their death with what he had recorded during his examination and treatment when they were alive. He found that lung restrictions and scarring led to tension around the organs. These lung issues could even lead to changes in the structure of bones in the neck and in the shape of the spine. These findings led Barral to the development of visceral evaluative techniques (known as Listening). Through this research he was also able to start putting together scientific findings supporting the bonesetter's organ manipulation and from there to document the relationships of the internal organs to one another and to the hard frame (bones), nerves, blood vessels, emotional links, and movement.

Along with his friend and colleague Pierre Mercier, Barral studied the movements of the organ system in three dimensions and learned how organs glide against each other with movement. The two men also studied the potential of the visceral (organ) system to promote lines of tension within the body, and the notion that tissues have memory. All this was fundamental to Barral's development of Visceral Manipulation, which in France is known as "liquid osteopathy."

With the help of Dr. Serge Cohen, a Grenoble radiologist, Barral documented changes in the viscera before and after manipulation. They employed X-ray fluoroscopy and ultrasound to record changes in position, motion, fluid exchange, and evacuation. Later, along with a team of electrical engineers and technicians they conducted additional research, studying infrared emissions from the body.

Now Barral has teamed up with Alain Croibier, a French osteopath, and they have expanded their ideas to include working on the nervous system, circulatory system, and joints. They have carried out research using techniques like Doppler scanning to prove the validity of their ideas, and have worked on tens of thousands of patients.

Jean-Pierre Barral was born in Grenoble, France, on September 25, 1944. He was a physiotherapist first, and then trained as an osteopath, earning his diploma in Osteopathic Medicine in 1974 from the European School of Osteopathy, in Maidstone, England. He went on to teach spinal biomechanics at the school from 1975 to1982. Through his background as a physiotherapist and osteopath, Barral approaches the body holistically. Therefore, until such time as every component of the human being has been addressed, new developments in VM seem likely.

Barral is a very humble man. He does not see himself as the inventor of Visceral Manipulation, but rather its developer. He sees his role as bringing science and validity to the concept of manipulating the organs and soft tissues, and to the recording techniques that he and his colleagues have found consistently reliable. Barral, in the interview mentioned above, says he is very proud of Visceral Manipulation and his contribution to it but that there are still so many things we don't know and that are not finished. He reports he feels proud because he can teach things to help patients—for him the results that can be achieved for the patient are primary. In his view, helping the patient feel better is his only goal. He describes himself as a real therapist and not only a teacher who teaches what he does in his office every day.

Visceral Manipulation is not usually taught in medical schools. Currently, in some European osteopathic schools VM comprises twenty-five percent of the exam content, something that Barral feels justly proud of. He certainly intends to continue working with and developing VM and in the video interview mentioned above states that he is "very anxious to do a little more; I am not satisfied because when you are, you are ready to die and I am certainly not ready to die." He is quoted elsewhere as saying "I prefer to die in the standing position" (i.e., at work). (*Natural Awakening,* September 2007.)

Barral has been teaching VM techniques since the 1980s in Europe, Asia, and the United States. Since then he has trained a team of international instructors, who teach Visceral Manipulation seminars to healthcare professionals around the world through the Barral Institute.

In 1999, in its feature "Innovators: *Time* 100—The Next Wave in Alternative Medicine," *Time* magazine (UK) listed Barral as one of the top one hundred to watch for in the new millennium. This is certainly a title he has earned and continues to earn.

3

# Healthcare Overview and Where Visceral Manipulation Fits In

In the Western world, healthcare is commonly divided into conventional and complementary medicine. Conventional healthcare is usually regarded as the domain occupied by medical doctors, nurses, occupational therapists, physiotherapists, midwives, psychologists, and others who work in the hospital environment. It tends to focus on prolonging our lives and addressing symptoms that make us feel unwell.

The focus of conventional medical care is generally to take responsibility for our health and "cure" whatever condition that we have. However, this is an attitude that is changing with time. As Barral states in the 2007 revision of his book *Visceral Manipulation II,* "The medical field is constantly evolving, and we are pleasantly surprised by the fact that mainstream doctors speak more and more of the ill patient rather than just the illness."

Conventional medicine tends to involve the use of drugs, surgery, and rehabilitative techniques. Its forte is its ability to save lives in cases of an accident or a life-threatening illness. However, many medical treatments do have side effects and in some cases do not address the underlying cause of an illness. For example, painkillers can help relieve pain but not treat the source of the pain. These treatments can be totally necessary for our survival and sanity, but sometimes they leave people searching for other solutions.

As Barral says, "Mainstream medicine is not the only medicine, and the patients have a need for all those alternative branches that can assist them. It should not be up to the medical doctors to decide who belongs and who does not; the patient is the only one who should decide that." *(Visceral Manipulation II.)*

Within the conventional medical world there are various specialties, each designed to address an area of dysfunction that can occur in the body. For example, cardiology addresses heart problems, while oncology addresses cancer and its effects. Complementary therapists tend to view the body more as a whole. They believe that it is impossible to isolate any body system, and that the whole body is interrelated and interdependent.

Complementary therapies are sometimes known as alternative therapies and occupy the second realm of today's healthcare. I would argue that they are not alternative, as I think both conventional and complementary approaches are essential. Indeed, if I were knocked down by a bus, I would want to be taken straight to a hospital to receive medical care—surgery to repair my broken bones and sew up my wounds, and medication to prevent infection and help me with my pain. However, if I had a headache and my doctor's only suggestion was to take painkillers, then I might investigate complementary therapies to help me identify the factors that have led to my symptoms. In my opinion, where conventional medicine excels is in acute care, providing essential surgery or medication. Complementary medicine, on the other hand, excels in improving quality of life—helping people get to the root of those everyday chronic challenges that wear them down.

There are many complementary therapies, including chiropractic, osteopathy, massage therapy, acupuncture, shiatsu, homeopathy, herbalism, CranioSacral therapy, kinesiology, and reflexology, to name but a few. These tend to focus on balancing the person as a whole by paying more attention to helping him or her achieve wellness, both physically and mentally, rather than addressing specific symptoms. Improving health often leads to the resolution of symptoms.

I believe that Visceral Manipulation crosses the boundaries between the conventional and complementary worlds. People from both worlds have trained in VM, and because it is a postgraduate training, they then incorporate it into their work. As a result, there are a large number of physiotherapists and medical doctors, as well as a large number of complementary therapists such as chiropractors, osteopaths, and massage therapists, who have trained in and use VM. Visceral Manipulation approaches the body in a holistic manner (looking at the body as a whole), so in some ways it could be classed as more on the complementary side. However, in its scientific approach it bridges both worlds, and may be used in conjunction with conventional medical or complementary approaches equally well.

## How is Visceral Manipulation Different?

Like many complementary therapies VM does not focus on symptom treatment, but rather on removing restrictions to allow a body to function optimally and health to improve. A VM practitioner will follow body tissue restrictions to determine the areas of dysfunction in a body. The area of restricted Mobility may not be anywhere near where the symptoms are. For example, a tissue pull in the belly may be the underlying cause of chronic back pain. Oftentimes, as a welcomed positive side effect of holistic treatment, long-term issues that a patient may not even have mentioned may also resolve with the treatment.

When considering an internal organ ailment, for example gallbladder problems, the conventional medical profession would probably recommend either medication or surgery. Complementary therapies might treat the gallbladder by working with it to improve its blood, nerve, or acupuncture meridian function, or use herbal or homeopathic treatments to address its problems.

Visceral Manipulation differs from conventional medicine in that the practitioner works on the restrictions in the body that are most prominent at the time of each therapy session; the process might involve working with an organ or its surrounding tissues. The practitioner usually considers the nerve and blood supply, and perhaps the emotional components associated with the organs.

Barral calls the gallbladder "a small pocketful of annoyance," as this is one of the first organs to react when a person becomes annoyed. So perhaps this emotional aspect is playing a part in the dysfunction. However, the gallbladder issue might be secondary to some other problem in the body, perhaps congestion in the intestines, so that might be the area that is treated. Visceral Manipulation follows the tissues to allow them to express what they need to release, and hence it often treats the parts that other therapies don't address. According to Barral, "We often get called in when regular medicine can't do anything, and that's where being an organ mechanic is a beautiful thing. There aren't many of us, and there are a lot of organisms out there that need help."

Visceral Manipulation is also used for problems or pain that appear to be unrelated to the internal organs. This is because VM is a broader treatment modality than simple manipulation of the internal organs. It also addresses nerves, blood vessels, and joints, for example. But in many cases, a problem that appears to be mechanical, of perhaps one joint, actually originates elsewhere in the body. It is the compensations for the original issue that have become symptomatic. Indeed, Barral has found that as much as ninety percent of all musculoskeletal problems have a visceral component. Musculoskeletal problems are issues with the muscles and bony frame of the body. He has found that over time a structural issue will start to affect the body's organs. For example, a dancer's hip problem may affect an organ such as the bladder, as the tissue tensions affect the internal pelvic contents. Or it may be that an organ has been the primary culprit leading to compensatory changes. So perhaps a bladder restriction has created tensions affecting the hip joint. Another example of organs affecting the musculoskeletal system is that people with asthma often end up with rib restrictions.

Visceral Manipulation can often be used to resolve pain that improves after manual therapy to the symptomatic area but then returns within a few weeks of the final session. If the primary pain is in the viscera and it has not been treated, the pain pattern resulting from it will recur until the primary issue in the organs has been resolved. In this way, VM is often used to break the cycle of a recurring symptom and allow its resolution. Additionally, any symptom can be due to a wide variety of causes. For this reason a person does not have to be suffering from symptoms related to organ dysfunction for the organs to be treated. Conversely, someone may have symptoms related to an organ and find that his or her practitioner treats an area that seems unrelated.

Conditions seemingly unrelated to the organs, but amenable to VM treatment are:

**ACUTE DISORDERS**

- Whiplash
- Seatbelt injuries
- Sports injuries

**MUSCULOSKELETAL DYSFUNCTION**

- Chronic spinal dysfunction
- Headaches and migraines
- Torticollis
- Carpal or tarsal tunnel syndrome
- Back, hip, knee, ankle, shoulder, elbow, and wrist pain
- Sciatica

**PAIN RELATED TO**

- Post-operative scar tissue
- Post-infection scar tissue

Throughout a VM session, both in the evaluative stage and during treatment, a practitioner will be *Listening* to the patient's body. Listening is a process of continuously feeling and following the specific tissue tensions that are within the body. It is only by following these tissue patterns that a practitioner can facilitate the body finding its own pathway to release. A fuller discussion about Listening appears later in this book, but this is really the art of VM.

This illustrates how VM is truly holistic. It addresses each component of possible dysfunction throughout the body in a totally individual manner as expressed by the body tissues. Visceral Manipulation practitioners focus not only on treatment of problems, but also on promotion of good health to prevent future issues. In *Understanding the Messages of Your Body,* Barral suggests that first of all, people should do everything they can do to stay healthy.

## Would Visceral Manipulation Be Used in Isolation or with Other Treatments?

Visceral Manipulation is taught only to those who have had previous healthcare training. For this reason, every practitioner has the option of using at least one other therapy with VM. Most practitioners will incorporate at least a few ideas from their other therapies with VM, although in some sessions they may use only VM evaluation and techniques. They really call upon their expertise to decide what is likely to bring about the best results for someone. For example, if that would be some stretching and the practitioner is a physiotherapist, he or she is likely to use physiotherapy techniques along with VM.

### *VM Gives Multiple Sclerosis Patient Back Her Quality of Life*

Agnes was a fifty-year-old woman who came to my clinic who had been diagnosed with multiple sclerosis and was complaining of various symptoms related to the disease. Multiple sclerosis (MS) is a condition that affects the nerves and nerve cells and can have widespread neurological ramifications. The conventional medical profession has no known cure for MS, and sufferers often turn to complementary therapies to help manage their symptoms. Agnes came to me about her difficulties walking. She had previously been to homeopathy and acupuncture, and while both helped a little with her energy levels and general feeling of well-being, she was still searching for ways to help improve her health.

With VM, I started off evaluating her body in the standing position to find the area of greatest restriction at that moment. This led me to her bladder area. I confirmed the restriction by checking Mobility of the bladder with its surrounding tissues. This revealed tightness and general fixation of the bladder. I checked the bladder's own intrinsic motion (known as Motility) and found this greatly reduced. I shared these findings with Agnes, and at this stage she told me she also suffered from urinary incontinence.

To help Agnes, I had her lie on her back. I started off releasing the ligaments in front of her bladder and then the pelvic floor. I also balanced her bladder with her sacrum (tailbone area), and then encouraged the Motility of her bladder to return more fully.

At her following session, Agnes came in walking a little easier than she had previously, although still with a slight limp. But from her perspective, the big success was that her bladder function had significantly improved, even though she had been unaware that this might be a benefit of the treatment. Before came to me she had only heard of my helping joint problems. This change in her bladder had been significant—she had gone from using the toilet every twenty to thirty minutes plus having several accidents per day to being able to wait for up to four hours. Previously her bladder had disrupted her life so much that she had rarely left her neighborhood. She was now able to go shopping in the city, which required a ferry ride from where she lived. As a result of this new-found freedom, her state of mind improved, and although she still had occasional incontinence with laughing or coughing, she felt she now had a greater quality of life. After meeting with her medical practitioner, she was able to stop using the patches she had used to control her bladder, and this relieved the dry-mouth issue that had been a side effect of the patches.

---

4

# The Philosophy Behind
# Visceral Manipulation

The human being is complex, composed of various parts that all work together harmoniously in health. These components are interrelated in ways that are almost impossible to comprehend. There are various levels of organization within the body, but many more that are still not understood. To help us comprehend the intricacies of the body, this chapter will discuss some of these levels of organization.

## The Systems Addressed by Visceral Manipulation

First we will look at the body from a systems perspective. To help us understand this, let's compare the human body to a car. While the body is not totally mechanistic like a car, I hope this analogy helps show how interrelated the components of the body are and how they can affect one another. However, we must remember that the softness and fluidity of the body does not exist in a machine.

A car in its finely tuned state runs perfectly, smoothly, and quietly. But with a small misalignment, a bug in the computer, or a sticking piston, a car is unable to function properly.

A human body and a car have many similar components. The structure of the car would be the chassis, the bodywork, the wheels, the engine, and so on. The structure of the human body would be the skeleton, muscles, ligaments, tendons, and organs.

In a car, if the wheels are not aligned and the steering wheel pulls to the right, the car is unlikely to function well. In our human body, if posture is out of balance, causing the lungs to have restrictions around them, inhibiting their normal motion and breathing ability, we do not work as well as we could.

Much of the activity in a modern car is governed by a central computer. In the human body, the brain, whose function includes emotional responses and the nervous system, is the governor. If there is a fault in the car's computer it can slow down and stop responding in a useful manner—likewise for the human body. The "fault" in the brain could be an old emotional response to a particular situation that was useful at one time but has now become outdated, or a glitch in the nervous system that means a person struggles to calm down his or her body after a stressful situation. Both a car and a human have a wiring system that allows communication to and from the central computer. In the human body it is known as the nervous system, which links our brain to all our body tissues—from the muscles in the big toes to the digestive system.

The car also has chemistry, which would be the water, oil, and fuels. These are carried in the car in pipes and hoses. Likewise, the human body has a chemical balance, consisting of the food and drink it takes in and the hormonal and blood systems. Did you know the average human body contains enough iron to make a 3-inch (8 cm) nail, enough sulphur to kill all the fleas on an average dog, and enough carbon to make nine hundred pencils? It also carries sufficient potassium to fire a toy cannon, enough fat to make seven bars of soap, enough phosphorous to make twenty-two hundred match heads, and water to fill a 10-gallon (45 l) tank. All of this creates a balance that is important for the body's functioning. If you put diesel into a gasoline-powered (petrol) car, it doesn't function well. Likewise, in the human body diet and fluid intake can greatly affect the tissues. In a car, if the gas (fuel) line gets restricted, it leads to poor running of the car. The same situation exists in the body if a blood vessel or tube in the digestive system is not functioning well—it can lead to big problems for the person.

So, what is the relevance of all this to VM? Visceral Manipulation considers all areas of the body to be interconnected, whether it's how the toe affects the neck or how the fluids and structure affect one another. A VM practitioner may consider the structure of your body, your nervous system, vascular or blood flow systems, emotional functioning, and also your lifestyle factors, such as diet or exercise. The pathway to health for you may be different than the pathway to health for another person. Visceral Manipulation is not about a set formula for "fixing problems." It is about finding the unique areas of restriction in the body that are inhibiting proper movement (and therefore function), then allowing the tissues to release in the unique way they need to so that the body can self-heal. This approach, which is congruent with Jean-Pierre Barral's osteopathic background, is expanded on in the next section.

## Basic Ideas from Which Visceral Manipulation Developed

As an osteopath, Jean Pierre-Barral based his work on the theories behind osteopathy, which were set forth in the late 1800s by the developer of osteopathy, Andrew Taylor Still. The theories are as follows:

1. The body is a unit—meaning the body functions as a whole, and a practitioner can't pass over any components when considering issues in the body. Consideration has to include structural problems, nervous system restrictions, emotional issues, hormonal or chemical imbalances, and so on, and then take into account how these impact one another and the body as a whole.

2. Structure and function are interrelated. This means that if there is a structural problem it will lead to impaired function, and vice versa. If someone has torn cartilage in a knee and can't bend it easily, this

will impact his or her functional ability to walk. Likewise, function-
ally, if someone walks in very high heels for much of her life, it is
likely to cause a structural change in her knee joint.

3. The body is a self-correcting and self-regulatory system—which
   means if you cut yourself you do not have to do anything for the
   cut to start healing. Additionally, this means that once a restriction
   has been removed, the body will automatically reorient itself toward
   health and better functioning.

4. Find it, fix it, and leave it alone. The aim of treatment is to find and
   address the main dysfunction in the body and then give the body
   time to self-correct. For this reason VM sessions will typically be
   scheduled with time in between for the body to adapt.

5. Rule of the artery is supreme. By this, Still meant that a lot of manual
   therapy should be focused on "irrigation of the withering fields," in
   other words, ensuring that there is adequate blood flow and therefore nutrition getting through to all the tissues. This will be discussed
   further in Chapter 11, "Circulation."

Given these basic principles that osteopathic medicine is based upon, it
is easy to see how Barral has developed these concepts and used them
as the foundation for VM.

## Components of Visceral Manipulation

Visceral Manipulation aims to gently restore the body to optimum structure and function. To identify areas of restriction and how they need
to be released, the practitioner will feel the tissues and their tensions.
As mentioned earlier, this is known as Listening and is one of the most
important tenets of VM. As each person is unique, only by following
an individual's body tensions can a practitioner best determine how to
help a particular body release.

Organs move in three dimensions; therefore, restrictions occur in three dimensions. Visceral Manipulation treatment aims to restore motion in all three planes of motion:

- Up and down
- Front to back
- Side to side

Through the capacity of VM to work with this harmonious approach, a body can resolve restrictions in the most efficient way and regain its self-healing capability.

If we take each of the components of the body discussed above in turn, we can see how VM addresses them. For structural problems, be these in the bony frame, soft tissues, or internal organs, the VM practitioner finds the point that causes the greatest restriction to movement or increases tension on the tissues, and releases this area. This in turn will allow the affected tissues and compensatory patterns to return to normal function. This is an example of structure governing function; in VM terms, this is known as the Mobility of the tissues.

Likewise, where an organ has a functional problem, a VM practitioner uses techniques to restore the normal intrinsic rhythm of the organ (known as Motility) and allow the function to normalize. Motility can be reduced by an issue within the organ itself, perhaps inflammation, emotional concerns, or in relation to medication. In these cases, Motility treatment restores the energy balance of the organ. Motility reduction may also be due to surrounding structures that have been binding an organ and impinging on its cellular motion. In these cases Motility treatment is used after Mobility release to remind the organ of its inherent motion pathway.

Where there is a problem with the nervous system, Jean-Pierre Barral, along with Alain Croibier, has developed a system for releasing nerve restrictions.

Where there is a chemical problem in terms of VM, the blood vessels (or hoses) can be released to allow improved circulation. These techniques are focused on allowing normal blood flow to the tissues, and it is this blood flow that allows nutrients to reach all parts of the body and waste products to be removed. It also helps oxygen to reach the tissues, without which life is not possible. Additionally, to address the chemistry, the practitioner may address lifestyle issues, suggesting, for example, dietary adjustments or exercise programs.

Through applying the theories outlined above, VM helps remove blockages and allows the body to heal itself. If there are no structural or functional problems, and the chemical balances are correct, then there is no reason why the body should not fully heal and become well.

## Visceral Reflexes

Between every vertebra of the spine, a pair of nerve roots leaves the spinal cord (one on each side) to supply areas of the body, skin and muscle. They are like telephone wires, both able to take messages to the areas they supply and bring back messages from those areas to the brain, via the spinal cord. Once the nerve moves away from the spine, it splits into branches. One of these goes to an area of skin, another to an area of muscle and another to an internal organ. As these branches are all connected. This means the body can get confused as to which of the branches has a problem or is being stimulated. When this happens a person may feel pain or suffer spasms in an area that actually has nothing wrong with it, but through confusion of this system is reflecting something from one of the other connected branches.

One of the best-known examples of this is someone with heart problems. It is common knowledge that if someone has a heart attack, that person often feels pain in the underside of the left arm. There is nothing wrong with this area of the arm; rather, it is supplied by the same nerve as supplies the heart. (See Figure 4.1.) The brain is not sure where the

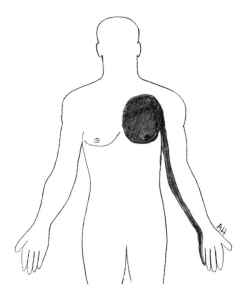

Figure 4.1. Area of skin
supplied by same nerves
as the heart

problem is, so it perceives both areas as painful. This phenomenon means that sometimes treating an organ with VM may be the key to relieving a pain somewhere else in the body, or conversely, a pain somewhere in the body may be indicative of an internal organ issue.

In similar fashion, there may be reflexes between two organs. Some nerve roots supply more than one organ, so if there is an issue with one, the other may become involved. For example, the pancreas and liver have some nerve supply in common, so both may be affected when a problem started with just one of them.

As the nerve roots come from the spine, a restriction at a level of the spine may lead to problems or pain in the organs, areas of skin, or muscle supplied from this level. An extreme example is the loss of muscle tone seen in the areas below a spinal cord injury after the injury. This phenomenon can also work in reverse; for example, a digestive problem can lead to restrictions of the vertebral levels that surround the associated nerve root. Because of their common nerve roots, bony restrictions can lead to pain or organ dysfunction, and conversely, organ dysfunction can lead to problems of the spine and muscles.

There is another nerve supply to many tissues, including all the internal organs, called the autonomic nervous system. It is divided into two parts, the sympathetic and parasympathetic systems. The sympathetic system is the one that deals with stress, making a person want either to fight or flee a stressful situation. The parasympathetic system is what calms us down once the situation has passed. These two systems need to be in balance for normal body functioning. However, in cases of prolonged stress, the continuous emotional stimulation of the sympathetic system may lead to a change in muscle tone, and so the emotional functioning can affect the body tissues. Likewise, if there is prolonged dysfunction of an organ, it may lead to altered autonomic nervous system tension, which in turn will be perceived as an emotional stress. So once again, this reflex works both ways.

The reflexes described above are why the symptoms that may change after Visceral Manipulation can seem so diverse and unrelated. It is also the reason that a person may receive treatment of an internal organ for a problem that he or she thought was a joint problem, perhaps a pain as far away from the organs as a toe or finger joint. These reflexes play a part in the consideration a VM practitioner makes when assessing and treating a patient's system.

## The Importance of Movement and Visceral Manipulation

Life requires movement. If there are restrictions in the body preventing movement then they will prevent optimum health. These movements can range from the smallest pulsing of an artery or a cell to the movements of the diaphragm (which allow us to breathe) up to the use of our arm that allows us to feed ourselves. When structures are restricted and affecting any one of the thousands of movements that happen daily in our body, our lives will be poorer as a result. Caroline Stone, DO, in her 2006 book, *Visceral and Obstetric Osteopathy,* goes so far as to say, "Assessing quality of motion is like assessing someone's quality of life:

poor movement not only indicates that the person is not able to physically live their lives to the full or express themselves with ease, but also that their body systems are not functioning optimally and that their health and immunity are compromised as a result."

The internal organs (viscera), muscles, ligaments, fascia, and blood vessels all move continuously. With breathing, the diaphragm moves 24,000 times per day; imagine how that increases if a person decides to go for a run. It is not just the diaphragm (a breathing muscle) that moves when one breathes. The lung tissue itself has to swell and contract with the volume of air. The rib cage that surrounds the lungs, and all the attached muscles, ligaments, and fascia must move freely for optimal function. Additionally, there are blood vessels that bring nutrients and nerve fibers that send signals to the cells that have to work to allow breathing to happen.

In breathing, movement is not limited to the chest area. The surrounding organs, the heart, liver, kidneys, spleen, stomach, and bowel are all directly affected by the movement of the chest. There are pulls through the connective tissues that mean there are probably very few cells that are not affected by the diaphragm's motion. This shows how interconnected all our parts really are! With each breath the kidneys will move up and down by around 4 inches (10 cm). In a lifetime they will move 19,000 miles (31,000 km)—that is just short of the distance around the earth (25,000 miles, which is 39,000 km). And on top of the up and down motion, the kidneys also have to rotate and move sideways. That is a lot of movement involved with just breathing.

Now imagine there is a restriction that stops the liver from moving properly with the diaphragm. The right lung will not be able to fully inflate and the rib cage on that side that cannot fully expand. The kidney, gallbladder, and bowel will be forced to move around the restricted area on the right side of the body. That restriction can perhaps lead to toxicity in the tissues because the liver cannot work properly, poor digestion because the gallbladder cannot squirt out its bile as effectively to help break down fat, pain from the restricted ribs, which may then affect the shoulder blade and arm function, and so on. So as the saying goes, "If you think you are too small to be effective, try lying in bed with a mosquito." The smallest restriction can lead to great discomfort or loss of function in the body.

It is not just the lungs that have motion. Every organ has its own intrinsic motion in three dimensions: the heart beats, blood vessels pulse, the bladder and bowel fill and empty. For women, there are menstrual cycles, pregnancy and delivery—and the pulsing of the fluid around the brain and spinal cord (craniosacral rhythm). There are also the voluntary movements—walking, stretching, running, swimming, dancing. All the organs and tissues have to be able to move when their surrounding structures move—if they didn't it wouldn't be long before we would tear or injure something. The tissues and organs need to be able to slide against and glide over each other in response to the movements that affect them. Visceral Manipulation aims to allow this freedom of motion to be restored.

## Lesional Chains

*Lesion* is the osteopathic term for a restriction of a tissue. A restriction in one part of the body does not remain isolated. Due to the interconnectedness of the body, the transmission of pressure, movement, posture, and tension rapidly cause the restriction in one tissue to lead to a whole series of compensations and changes in other tissues of the body. So where the problem starts off in the big toe, this changes the dynamics of the foot and ankle, which affects how we walk, leading to pelvic imbalances. These in turn may lead to changes in the functioning of the pelvic organs, perhaps leading to constipation or abdominal pain, or changes in the spine leading to neck pain or headaches. A person may experience neck pain and headaches, and the actual cause could be from the big toe. This is what is known as a lesional chain—the chain of reactions set off by one restriction or lesion. In many cases a lesional chain may not have any symptoms, as the body is still able to compensate for the pattern of tension. But over time, the body is less able to compensate, and symptoms begin to appear. Lesional chains explain why a practitioner can seem to be addressing parts of the body unrelated to the symptoms.

In VM a practitioner will aim to find the start of the lesional chain, and helping to normalize that area may well resolve a number of residual problems that a restriction had caused. By Listening to the tissues, meaning feeling for and following restrictions, a practitioner is able to find the primary problem to address. Jean-Pierre Barral often quotes Rolin Becker, another osteopath, in saying "only the tissues know."

Visceral Manipulation is about your practitioner Listening, feeling, and following your tissues to help your body find its own pathway to health. In the next few chapters we will discuss how practitioners discover where the main issue is in the body and the treatment they might give.

### Wide Range of Symptoms Developed Two Years after Car Accident

Hamish retired early due to various health concerns that seemed to have developed over the prior two years. He reported that he had suffered a whiplash injury two years ago from an accident in which a car skidded on ice. In the months following the accident, other than having some neck pain, he had felt well. However, various seemingly unexplainable health concerns had developed since that time, and his anxiety levels led to him taking early retirement.

Hamish suffered from neck pain, headaches, chest pain, tiredness, episodes of feeling his heartbeat going very fast, digestive sluggishness, constipation, and at times, feeling he could not catch his breath properly. The diagnosis of his general practitioner was that Hamish was suffering from anxiety attacks.

Visceral Manipulation evaluative techniques took me to Hamish's chest area, specifically his breastbone (sternum), and from there into his right chest and pleura (membrane bag that contains the lung). A ligament that attaches to the lung on the right side (pulmonary ligament) showed itself to be the primary restriction in his body.

I applied treatment to this ligament and the ligament that runs between the two collarbones across the top of the sternum (the interclavicular ligament). Then I released his sternomanubrial joint (joint between the upper and lower parts of the breastbone), as well as the tissue (pleura) surrounding his right lung. I finished up balancing the Motility of his two lungs with one another.

When Hamish returned a month later, his evaluation led to the left triangular ligament of the liver. I treated this with him in a seated position, and combined the treatment with movements of his right arm to help the release.

By his third session, less than two months after his initial presentation, he reported that all his symptoms had resolved, but he questioned whether they could all really have been related to his car accident. His accident had been two years ago, and he was surprised that if it had really caused all his problems, his symptoms had not started immediately following it. He said some of them had even taken a year or more to develop. This led me to explain how interconnected the body is and how over time unresolved tensions lead to more problems. I suggested that perhaps his sternum and right lung area had been compressed during the accident by his seatbelt (in Scotland the driver sits on the right of the car, so the seatbelt would have crossed his right shoulder). This could have led to the lung restrictions and hence the breathing difficulties. The pericardium, the membrane bag that surrounds the heart, connects in behind the sternum, so it could have been affected by the ongoing restriction, leading to his rapid heart beats. And his headaches and neck pain may have been due to the whiplash, or perhaps due to the pull on the fascia from the restrictions in his chest area.

The liver often is affected by trauma, as the shock waves are transmitted through the tissues, and the liver is large and fairly solid and has the weight of the heart above it. This may be the reason that once the restrictions in his chest were resolved, the liver showed as being the main concern of Hamish's body. Perhaps this led to the digestive sluggishness and constipation over time, as the liver was not functioning optimally. Alternatively, the problems could have been the effects on the nervous system or blood flow to the digestive organs, as both run through the chest area. This, along with his breathing and pain issues, would inevitably lead to tiredness. His anxiety increased as a result of not understanding why these seemingly random symptoms developed. These explanations are only one possibility for Hamish's symptoms. As the interconnectedness of the body is so intricate, there may have been other compensations that created these same symptoms.

5

# Visceral Manipulation Evaluation Techniques—How Does Your Practitioner Decide Where to Treat?

Your VM practitioner will evaluate your body for areas of tension, rather than areas of symptoms. A restriction is an area of reduced flexibility that will pull the surrounding tissue toward it, and your practitioner will feel this under his or her hand. This helps find the area that your body is most concerned with at the time of your exam. This area may or may not be where you are experiencing symptoms. As we discussed in an earlier chapter, this is because the core, or primary, tension causes compensatory patterns in your body. It is these patterns that may cause the pain and reduction in movement you are experiencing. We do not feel much of what is going on in our organs, otherwise we would feel each thing we ate on its entire digestive journey. So for an organ to give us pain there has to be a more severe restriction and something has to have caused swelling, inflammation, or congestion. For this reason you may not actually know you have an issue with the organ that turns out to be the primary trigger for your symptoms. For greatest efficiency and best results, if your practitioner addresses your primary tension, it will allow resolution of your compensatory patterns and therefore your symptoms. Visceral Manipulation considers any possible part of the body or type of restriction, as it is a holistic approach.

Practitioners of VM are trained to feel where the tensions are in the body. Using their anatomical knowledge along with their skilled hands they are able to determine which structures are affected and how best to work with them to allow release. This is known as Listening, a term touched on earlier. It is a term used by well-known osteopath Rollin Becker, which Jean-Pierre Barral uses because he feels "this admirable word conveys the modesty and gentleness which [you] the practitioner should manifest." (*Visceral Manipulation I,* 1988.) Listening is indeed an art. It is used in Visceral Manipulation to help your practitioner evaluate your body and to discover its pathway to health. It is used not only to guide your practitioner to what needs treating, but also throughout each treatment session to allow the practitioner to best feel how your tissues need to be released.

The majority of the VM evaluation techniques are done with your practitioner's hand. Jean-Pierre Barral says "I try to feel. I try to know what kind of messages the body sends to me … I am a hand worker, when I see people doing massage with a machine, I am surprised because there is connection somewhere, when you put your hand on somebody." (*Natural Awakening,* September 2007.) The connection is what can make the treatment successful or not. According to Barral, "Sense is important … what you feel, see, smell; when I see somebody, I let the person come into my eyes. If you let someone come into you, it is different, you feel part of the person come to you.…" (Quoted by Kendra L. Arnold, in *Natural Awakening,* September 2007.)

At your initial meeting, your practitioner will already be noting details about how your body is functioning. It is actually many practitioners' preference to feel your body first, before hearing about your symptoms, so as not to be distracted from what your body tissues are actually trying to tell them. In a 2008 symposium, Barral explained, "I prefer to speak to the tissues not so much the person." This is because the primary tension may be in a location far removed from the site of symptoms. Your practitioner will also ask you about your symptoms and medical history before treatment commences. The assessment protocol outlined below may or may not be done in full, depending on the results of each step. The procedures described here may be included in an assessment.

## General Listening (GL)

General Listening begins the VM evaluation. Barral describes it as "receiving a message" and regards it as key to the effectiveness of VM. It leads your practitioner to *where* the primary restriction is in your body at that time and in that posture. This tells your practitioner where your body needs attention first to allow it to take its pathway to health. When possible the Listening is done while you are in a standing position with your practitioner positioned directly behind you. (See Figures 5.1 and

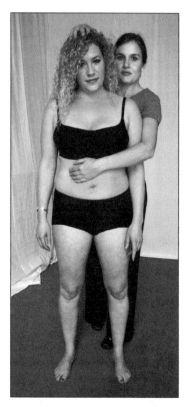

5.2.) Your practitioner then places one hand on the top of your head with the intention of collecting information about your entire body. He or she may ask you to close your eyes, to prevent you from stabilizing your body by focusing on an object. The practitioner wants your body to be able to truly express its pattern of restrictions. You may or may not find that you move slightly into a pattern, perhaps moving slightly to one side, forward or backward. This is an instance where "the body hugs the lesion," meaning, your body hugs its restriction.

Figure 5.1. General Listening
(view from the front)

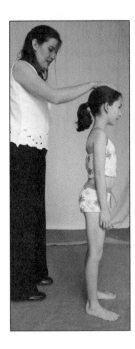

Figure 5.2. General Listening (view from the side)

The idea of your body hugging its restriction is not difficult to understand. You only need to think of the situation where someone is hit
hard in the stomach by a ball. Instantly the person's response is to grab
the area and bend forward and round it to take off the tension. This is
exactly the same response that your body tissues have, on a much more
subtle level. Additionally, through the interconnectedness of the fascia,
ligaments, tendons, organs, and muscles of your body, your practitioner
is able to feel where your body tensions pull to. The center of the pull
is the location of the tension your body is aware of at that time. Your
practitioner will gather information about whether the tension is more
toward the front of your body (possibly an internal organ), the back of
your body (maybe spinal), to one side or other (possibly a rib), and in
the upper or lower parts of your body.

## Manual Thermal Evaluation (MTE)

Manual Thermal Evaluation is based on the premise that there are temperature differences between normal and restricted tissues. Research carried out by Jean-Pierre Barral shows that this technique can be extremely accurate. Barral felt the bodies of patients just before they went into surgery or had a scan, and once they were opened up or scanned he was able to see exactly what and where the tension was. With experience he was able to precisely find and describe the issue before the skin was cut or the scan performed. In France, substantial research money has been put into Barral's MTE, leading to the development of an instrument called the "Orthoscan," which validates and duplicates the results of MTE. It has been found that the trained practitioner's hand can detect temperature differences of 1/20 degree Fahrenheit (1/10 degree Celsius).

You are probably already aware that areas with problems have different temperatures. If you hurt your ankle it will often feel hot, and the recommended treatment for a new injury often includes the use of ice to combat this heat. It is the same types of reaction that practitioners of VM are taught to feel for and include in their analyses.

Manual Thermal Evaluation is done with you lying on your back and your practitioner's hand moving in the air above you. (See Figure 5.3.) It may be done at two different levels—about 4 inches (10 cm) above your body gives information about your tissues, while around 12 inches (30 cm) from your body tells more regarding emotional issues. The distances allow your practitioner to feel the temperature differences in your body and find areas where the temperature diverges from the surrounding tissue. This is another indication of which area in your body is restricted and helps further pinpoint the best place for treatment to begin. Your practitioner will often scan over your whole body and limbs to check for any restrictions.

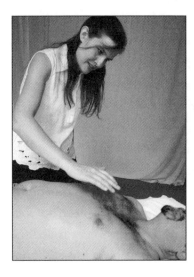

Figure 5.3. Manual Thermal Evaluation

## Local Listening

Local Listening is used to find precisely *what* anatomical structure your practitioner's hand was attracted to in the General Listening. At the area shown by the General Listening—a quadrant of the abdomen, an area of the chest, the skull, a leg, or an arm, your practitioner places a hand gently on your body and allows the tissues to attract the hand to the specific area of restriction. An area of the body that has lost proper Mobility movement will pull the surrounding tissue toward it, and this can be felt mechanically under their hand, as a Listening.

On some occasions the body requires a gentle nudge over a suspected area to "wake up" the tissues. In this case a gentle pressure is applied and then released to allow your practitioner to feel the pull in your tissues. This process is known as Active Listening, whereas the above process, without the gentle nudge, is known as Passive Listening.

Once an area of tension has been identified by Local Listening, your practitioner may use a technique called *Inhibition.* This is done by placing a gentle pressure on the restriction that supports the tissue temporarily both mechanically and through nerve reflexes. (See Figure 5.4.)

Your practitioner uses this to confirm he or she has found the precise location of your restriction.

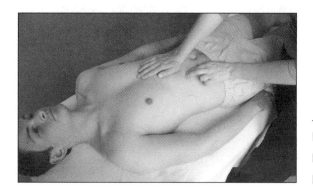

Figure 5.4. Local Listening with Inhibition

After the precise location of the tension has been identified your practitioner will place a hand on that structure to find out more about the exact nature of the restriction. He or she will be feeling whether the restricted site is limited in its scope to only affecting the local area or if it extends to more of the surrounding tissues, possibly involving other organs or structures (technique known as Extended Listening).

## Mobility

Mobility is the term used to describe how movable a structure is relative to the surrounding tissues. No part of your body exists in isolation, with every tissue or even every cell in your body being dependent on those around it for support and movement. Your tissues should be able to articulate with each other, and have good slide and glide (that is, ability for the organs to move freely against one another) with adjacent tissues and muscles. For example, the liver should be able to move easily in relationship to the diaphragm and the stomach. Mobility tests involve your practitioner gently moving a tissue in different directions against the tissues around it to find out if it has enough movement, stretch and support from the surrounding structures. (See Figure 5.5.) There may be one direction in which the tissue does not move as easily or smoothly as it should. The tissue will not stretch away from the exact point of the restriction. Alternatively, your tissues may be too lax, or slack, and may move too easily in one direction, indicating a structural injury or change. The changes in Mobility may or may not be something of which you are aware. For example, in order for you to bend forward, your internal organs must be able to slide and glide over one another. If they have reduced Mobility and can't move out of the way as they normally would, the body will over-compress its internal organ anatomy. As a result you may not be able to bend far enough to touch your toes.

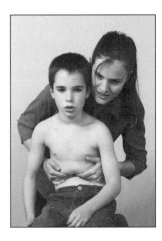

Figure 5.5. Mobility testing of the liver

## Leg Length Evaluation

Your practitioner may compare the length of your legs (or the lengths of your outstretched arms). He or she is looking to see if one side is pulled in toward the body due to a tension pattern within the tissues. It is very unusual to have a true (known as anatomical) difference in limb length unless there is a history of an accident, surgery, or infection to one side. More often, the difference in limb length is from one side being pulled into the body due to tension in the tissues. These cases they will often resolve within the treatment session.

## Tension Tests

There are various tension tests that your VM practitioner may use. These include the Lasegue, the Glenohumeral , and the Adson-Wright Articulation tests. (See Figure 5.6.) These involve your practitioner moving either your arm or leg into a particular position and checking for various responses, such as a change in pulse, symptoms, how easily it moves, or unusual movement patterns. Your practitioner then may hold areas of your body to see if they cause a change when the test is repeated, and this may show him or her how that area is affecting another or causing symptoms. Often practitioners will repeat the tests after they have treated you to see the results of the treatment.

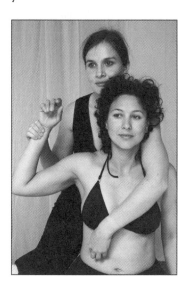

Figure 5.6. Adson-Wright tension test

## Skin Testing

The skin is the largest organ in the body, covering 20 square feet (1.9 sq m) in an adult man. There are 45 miles (72 km) of nerves in the skin of a human being, and each square inch (6 sq cm) of human skin consists of 20 feet (6 m) of blood vessels. Due to nerve and vascular (circulation) reflexes from the organs and body tissues, the area of skin overlying the problem in your body will feel thicker and have less elasticity (stretch). Practitioners will usually feel the skin between their fingers with a rolling action. This test simply indicates to them that they are over an area where there is an issue, but does not tell them what structure is affected. Having found the area, or used the technique to confirm other findings, practitioners will then use their Listening skills to accurately determine which structure is affected.

## Motility

Motility is a very subtle inherent tissue motion perceptible by the trained hand. Motility reflects the energetic cellular activity of an organ. This motion retraces the pathway of embryological migration of the organs, which was the pathway they followed during a person's development in the womb as the organs moved away from the midline of the body. For this reason the practitioner's hand feels Motility as a motion away from the midline and then back toward the midline of the body. These phases are termed *Inspir* and *Expir* (nothing to do with breathing) respectively and occur at the rate of about seven to eight cycles per minute.

Motility evaluation will usually be done after Local Listening on the specific organ identified. Your practitioner will assess Motility by placing just the weight of a hand over the organ. (See Figure 5.7.) Motility evaluates the vitality of an organ, meaning that an organ in good health goes easily into both Inspir and Expir. Inspir and Expir are evaluated for their frequency, rate (the ideal rate is about four seconds for each phase), quality (how smooth or uneven it feels), amplitude (how far it goes in each phase), and direction of the movement of your Motility (an organ in a state of equilibrium moves in three dimensions). Additionally, where there is a pair of organs in the body (like lungs or kidneys), the rhythm should be the same.

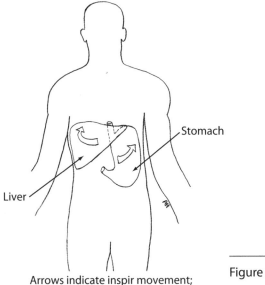

Arrows indicate inspir movement;
expir is opposite of arrows

Figure 5.7. Motility of liver
and stomach

## Emotional Listening

Your body tissues store emotional reactions—I am sure we have all had "butterflies in our stomach" or felt something "in our gut." However, these reactions can sometimes become more long-term serious problems for your body and can either lead to or result from organ dysfunction. You only have to enter a room with an angry person, and before they express themselves verbally you can already sense their emotion. Your trained VM practitioner is able to pick up on and evaluate such reactions and feel them coming from your tissues when there is an emotional component to your problems.

Typically, your practitioner will include the emotional evaluation at the same time as the evaluative procedures outlined above. For ease of understanding I am outlining the emotional component evaluation separately. The first step your practitioner will take is General Listening, sometimes with a very light pressure as he or she picks up electromagnetic disturbances in your body. With General Listening you may fall in a particular way that will give the practitioner a clue to your emotional state. For example, you may fall backward, which denotes an issue from your past that you are preoccupied with; you may fall forward, for an issue relating to your future. Falling to the left usually relates to more of a social issue, while falling to the right points to a personal concern. Falling also gives a clue to the organs affected, as hollow organs such as the gallbladder, stomach, duodenum, and small intestine relate more to falling to the left, along with social or relationship issues. Solid organs such as the liver, kidney, lung, and pancreas relate to personal issues, such as who you really are or your deep self.

Then your practitioner identifies which organ or part of your body the emotion is affecting. This is often done using Manual Thermal Evaluation. Emotional issues will affect the temperature farther away from the body than physical restrictions will, and are vaguer in size and shape. Your practitioner will feel at about 4 inches (10 cm) and then possibly move to about 12 inches (30 cm) from your body for these issues. Additionally, there are specific areas of your brain that relate to emotional issues. When there is an emotional component these will be activated and detectable to your practitioner, who will feel temperature changes from these areas.

## Other Evaluative Techniques That May Be Used in Conjunction with Visceral Manipulation

The techniques below may be used to help your practitioner gain more specific information regarding your health.

### Blood Pressure

Visceral Manipulation practitioners may take your blood pressure, often on both sides and possibly in your arms and legs, to compare your blood pressure from side to side and between limbs. Ideally, it should be equal all around. Where there is a restriction in one location or in only your upper or lower body, it may affect your blood vessels and the tissues around them, giving yet another clue to your practitioner as to where the tensions are in your body. Jean-Pierre Barral has found through observation of blood pressure in several thousand patients that there can be differences of 10 mm Hg (the unit used to measure blood pressure) or more, which often resolve with treatment of the affected areas with VM.

You may not have any symptoms of reduced blood pressure in one part of your body, or you may be aware something is not quite right. For example, you may find that one limb is always cold, and this could be due to reduced blood pressure to this limb. Receiving VM treatment may help your circulation and resolve your symptoms. For many people the blood pressure changes are so subtle that they may not be aware of any symptoms. However, the clues these changes give the practitioner can be valuable in determining where restrictions are in the body.

There can be numerous causes of unequal blood pressure, many of which might surprise you. These include a change in the tissues of a limb, for example, from trauma such as a sprain, break, or dislocation. Certain lung injuries can also result in blood pressure changes from one side to the other, as can neck injuries or arthritis. Internal organ restrictions are another cause of unequal blood pressure readings. It's thought that the reason for this is in the nervous system, as the affected organs give altered stimulus via nerves from the organ to the artery blood vessels walls. This changes the muscular tone of the arteries and therefore the blood pressure. After treatment, your blood pressure should become more equal. This is an indication to practitioners that they have worked on the correct area and their treatment has been effective.

Visceral Manipulation can make a difference in some cases of high blood pressure. Your kidneys are very much involved in blood pressure regulation, and if they are part of your problem, having treatment to release restrictions there may help reduce your blood pressure.

*Pulse*

Your practitioner may take your pulse in various parts of your body. Finding areas where it is harder to feel your pulse gives your practitioner a clue as to where there is restricted blood flow. As with blood pressure, it is possible that you will know that you have a problem with circulation to that area, although you also may be unaware of it. If circulation is restricted, it can reduce the blood that reaches certain areas. It is like not watering part of your garden—that part of it is unlikely to thrive or be as healthy as the part that is regularly irrigated. Lack of circulation can then lead to malfunctioning of the areas that are supplied by that blood vessel. For further information on blood flow issues, see Chapter Eleven, "Circulation."

While your therapist is feeling your pulse he or she may move part of your body or ask you to move something. By doing this, the practitioner can see if your pulse changes. If it does, it gives clues as to where your restrictions are and what is needed to help you.

## Differentiating between Types of Tissue

The art of VM is the sensitivity practitioners have developed in their hands to allow them to specifically feel different types of tissue and be able to accurately distinguish them. Just as a wine aficionado has developed the ability to taste the many subtleties of wine, a trained practitioner can feel the many subtleties of the tissues.

Some of these distinguishing features are listed below:

- Bone—Very hard, with very little stretch or give.

- Viscera (internal organs)—Having various different textures, depending on their makeup and function. All organs have a certain tone to them. Some organs are hollow, like the digestive tract or bladder. Others, like the liver or kidney, are more solid.

It is also possible to feel if the organ is muscular, like the heart or duodenum. Some organs are more fragile and softer, like the pancreas. Through very gentle palpation, VM practitioners learn to identify the specific qualities of each organ.

- Nerve—Firm, round, or oval, with a string-like feel. It is usually somewhat mobile and has some resistance to pressure. It may feel a little "buzzy" to your practitioner.

- Ligament—A thickened area of fascia that is flat, smooth, and attaches two structures.

- Tendon—Firm, and attaches to a muscle. It will change tension when a muscle is moved and tends to be more mobile than a nerve.

- Muscle—Less firm than a tendon or nerve. Changes diameter when it contracts or relaxes.

- Fascia—Flat, thin, smooth, sheet-like material.

- Septum—Found between muscles, generally, and is a thickened area of fascia. Tends to be larger and thicker than a nerve.

- Nerve ganglion (junction point of nerves)—Round and small, and a little less firm than a nerve. Should be mobile.

- Artery—More supple than a nerve—and pulses!

- Vein—Soft and flat, distensible.

- Lymph nodes—Nodes are round but irregularly shaped and give on touch.

The VM practitioner confirms the area shown by the General and Local Listening with Mobility testing. Put another way, the zone the practitioner was attracted to by the Local Listening will be restricted in its Mobility. It is through direct palpation, anatomical knowledge, and Mobility testing that the practitioner chooses the best treatment option for the specific anatomy involved.

## The Next Step

While these evaluative techniques will often be used to begin your VM session, they may be repeated during the session or at the end to assess results from the treatment. Your practitioner will be looking for changes from the initial findings and then allowing these changes to work through your tissues over the days or weeks following the treatment. This is the body self-correcting.

It needs to be noted at this point that it is not possible to identify every health issue by touch alone. So there may be occasions where a practitioner suggests further imaging or medical testing to help clarify a situation prior to treatment. Visceral Manipulation is to be used alongside conventional medical testing and care rather than as a blanket replacement for it. Your practitioner will advise you if further investigation or other care is required for your health.

To assist you in understanding how the various evaluative techniques are used during a VM session, the techniques are italicized in the patient case below.

### Bringing It All Together—A Case Story

Cara was a forty-five-year-old woman who came to see me for her right knee pain, which had started up gradually and would come and go for no apparent reason. She reported that it had bothered her on and off for years. She was not aware of any injury and couldn't pinpoint an exact time that the pain started.

Using *General Listening,* I was taken to Cara's right groin area. I followed up with *Manual Thermal Evaluation,* which also revealed a hot spot in the lower abdomen on the right but really no change in temperature over her knee area. I also found a warm spot on the right side at the area of the lower ribs. Using *Local Listening,* my hand was attracted by the tissues to her right lower abdomen and was aware of various pulls that seemed to radiate out from the scar of where her appendix had been removed ten years previously. With *Extended Listening,* I could feel that there were tensions that pulled to both the cecum (the first part of the large intestine) and the right ovary.

I Mobility tested her right knee but could find no restriction of the joint movement; the only finding I had around the knee was that she could feel the pain when I pressed various locations just above the joint. I then went on to *Local Listen* and *Mobility test* the cecum. I found that it felt pulled down and pulled toward the midline of her body. I could feel a tension that felt like a cord pulling in the same direction, which from my experience of different *tissue types* I knew was a ligament. Combined with my *anatomical knowledge* I realized this was her ligament of Cleyet, a ligament found in about sixty percent of women that attaches the cecum of the large bowel to the right ovary. My *anatomical knowledge* told me that this ligament crosses the femoral nerve that goes to the leg and supplies the knee area. Because of the tension I found, it seemed to me that the ligament could be compressing the nerve and causing her knee pain, which would not have needed a known accident to cause it. Using a *Motility assessment* I noted her right ovary seemed to have little Motility, which helped confirm my theory. There was no significant restriction of the colon Motility.

When I discussed my findings with Cara she then shared with me that she also had a lot of pain with her menstruation, especially on the right side. I told her of my hypothesis that it might have been aggravated by her appendix removal, and she said that she was sure that she had not had knee pain prior to that time. Also, her periods had seemed worse in the past few years.

I treated Cara six times at three- to four-week intervals. The treatment was focused on releasing the tension from the appendix scar and the effects of the scar on the ligament of Cleyet and the associated organs and femoral nerve. After two sessions her right knee pain resolved. By the sixth session she told me her periods were no longer painful. She was now having to look at the calendar to work out when her period was coming—a new experience, as usually pain for a few days leading up to it had signaled its impending arrival. She also reported having more energy, and no longer having a dull ache in her low back and pelvic area. Her skin was also improving, perhaps indicating a general improvement in her health as her body became more balanced.

# 6

# Treatment

Once the area requiring help has been identified, the practitioner has to find the exact structure involved. Supposing the area identified is the navel. Underneath the navel are multiple layers of tissues. From front to back, some of these tissues include: the skin; a layer of fat; a muscular layer; the peritoneum (thin membrane); ligaments called the ligamentum teres, which connects to the liver, and urachus, which attaches to the upper bladder; a fatty layer called the greater omentum, which is attached to the stomach; small intestines, which attach to the back; the duodenum; lots of fascia, arteries, veins and nerves; the bony vertebra and the spinal cord and its coverings; more muscle and finally, more fat and skin. (See Figure 6.1.) This means that once the area that is affected has been traced to your navel, the practitioner then needs to use their skills and knowledge to feel exactly which structure is affected.

When teaching, Barral has a mantra that he uses regularly: "Know your anatomy." He says that to this day he studies anatomy for at least two hours per week, as he has done for forty-plus years. It is only with anatomical knowledge that practitioners can know what structures could be affected under their hands.

Barral also regularly tells his students, "What we like is to be precise." He has found that by working with precision the treatment is more effective, requires less pressure, is not stressful to the body—and the results are faster. Being precise allows the intelligence of the tissues to find a way

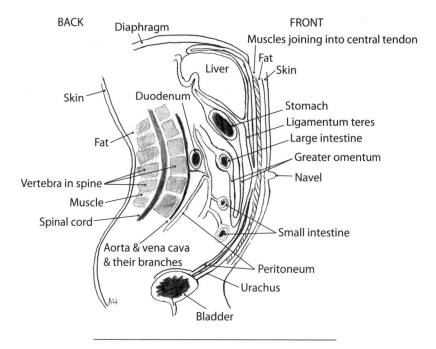

Figure 6.1. Layers of the body under the navel

to release. If an area of the body has not been able to move freely, there is a reduction in the nerve information being carried to the brain, and the body is less able to self-correct. Therefore, if an area that has been affected is stimulated even just a little, but very precisely, the body's own self-correcting ability will respond. A precise stimulus to the restricted area triggers the sending of a precise message to the brain. In return, the message sent from the brain on how the body needs to self-correct will be more precise. This means that practitioners will combine their anatomical knowledge with their hand skills to feel how far into a body the tension is, and the exact structure that is involved. Is it solid like a kidney, a flat surface like fascia, a round tube like a hollow organ or a vessel? These are just some of the questions practitioners may consider as they feel a body at a specific location to find the structure that needs some help to release.

Often someone comments, "All I came in with was a pain in my side, but now you are treating my belly button." Perhaps the pain in the person's side was due to the pull of the ligamentum teres, a ligament attached to the liver that was then pulling on the diaphragm (which lies above the liver) and was causing the pain. If the patient's diaphragm was released and nothing else, within hours, due to the ongoing pull of the ligament from the liver, the pain would return. However, if the ligament was released, the liver would no longer be pulled, which would then allow the diaphragm to relax, and the pain to resolve. Practitioners may end up treating a long way from a symptom but by following what they are feeling, they end up being more effective. Indeed, if all that needed to happen to resolve any pain was to rub over the local area, there would be little need for healthcare. Human bodies are so much more intricate and interconnected.

Once the exact structure has been identified, treatment can begin. Often treatment in VM is relatively quick compared to the evaluation process. The structure is found, and depending on what it is, various techniques can be used. The goal of treatment is to allow the structure to move and glide easily with its surrounding tissues and allow it to regain its own smooth, intrinsic motion, known as Motility. Jean-Pierre Barral and Pierre Mercier, in their 1988 book *Visceral Manipulation,* state that "We manipulate to the point where the body can take over in order to achieve self-correction, not to force a correction on the body." Visceral Manipulation is very much about allowing your body to heal itself and simply offering it a helping hand along the way.

Most VM treatment techniques are hands on the body. Usually the finger pads are used to gently feel through the body layers and reach the affected tissues. Throughout each technique practitioners will be feeling the body's tissues and how they are reacting and changing. With this information they will then be modifying their precise pressure to allow the body to release the most easily and fully in three dimensions. Each person and every restriction will have its own unique pathway to health. As Barral has instructed, "we need to follow the tissues, for they are better guides than our own reasoning." The most common treatment techniques are outlined below.

## Direction of Ease
## (Known as Indirect Techniques in North America)

Direction of ease techniques are often done first. To start this technique, a practitioner may use a gentle compression and release to the area a couple of times to "wake up" the tissues. Then he or she will use the sensitivity of the hands to follow the tissue in the direction it wants to go, and add very gentle encouragement (known as Induction) to allow it to move freely in that direction. The body's tissues usually know the easiest way to release. Direction of ease techniques give them the opportunity to find their own path without any stress being placed on them. This technique is often all that is required for them to be able to release their restrictions and is therefore easy on your body.

## Direct Stretch
## (Known as Direct Techniques in North America)

This is done by finding the affected structure and then following the tissues to the point of tension (or stretch). (See Figure 6.2.) The tension is often followed and held in a three-dimensional fashion, known as *stacking*. It is almost as if the tension is increased so much it draws the body's attention to it, and the body can then discover how much it is being affected and then start to release. As the tissues release, any extra slack is taken up, and the tissue followed until the tension disperses. This is usually done and held for up to forty seconds before pressure will be released a little, and then possibly repeated until the treatment of this area is complete. Alternatively, a practitioner will use a more rapid, oscillating motion to aid a direct stretch technique. A gentle stretch may be used to encourage shearing and gliding between two structures, or to stretch along the fiber orientation of a restricted tissue.

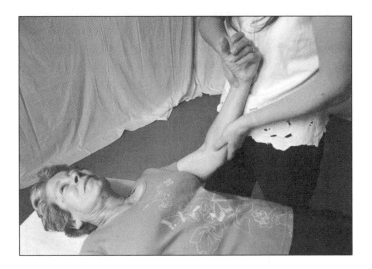

Figure 6.2. Direct stretch technique

## Line of Tension

When two or more organs or tissues are involved in the same restriction there can be a "line of tension" between them. Effectively resolving the restriction involves getting the tissues to "talk" with one another and sort out their issues. This can be either done as a direct stretch technique or a direction of ease technique.

## Long Levers

Sometimes, to help a release, practitioners may move the body or a limb or ask the patient to do this. For example, they may move one leg or ask a person to turn his or her head. (See Figure 6.3.) This can alter the tension around the restriction and encourage release in the tissues. It may also help bring in any elements of the restriction that are affecting more distant parts of the body, perhaps via a lesional chain.

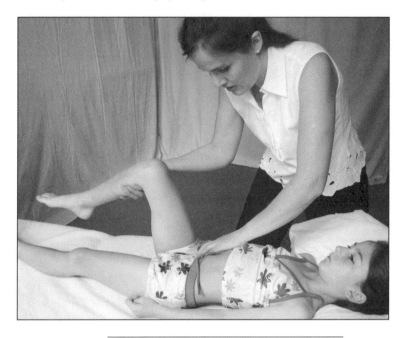

Figure 6.3. Using the right leg as a long lever

## Combined Technique

When a combination of direct stretch and long lever techniques is used, it is known as a Combined Technique. It can speed up and allow a deeper direct release.

## Recoil

This is a less-used technique and often reserved for a situation where other treatment methods are not resolving the issue or where a tissue is "frozen," meaning that an organ has lost its own intrinsic Motility.

Recoil is also often used when speed has been a factor in the formation of a restriction. For example, a patient may have been in a car accident, or even may simply say, "I suddenly coughed." The practitioner gathers up the affected structure and then springs back out of it to "wake up the tissues." (See Figure 6.4.) This focuses the attention of the body on this area, and stimulates the nervous system and blood vascular systems. It also seems to energize the area. It may be done on the start of breathing in and is sometimes repeated three to five times.

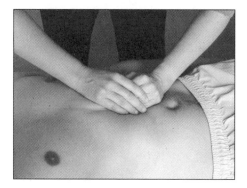

Figure 6.4. Using Recoil
on the left kidney

## Skin Rolling

Barral found that stimulation of the skin by rolling it between thumb and fingers can help either start or complete a release in the structures it over-lies. (See Figure 6.5.) This is thought to be due to the high nerve supply of skin, and the nerve reflexes that go into the deeper structures and organs. It is also used with nerve and vascular manipulation techniques.

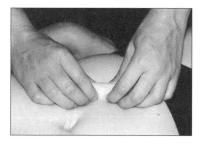

Figure 6.5. Skin rolling technique

## Treating Another Structure to Affect an Organ (European Definition of Indirect)

In this case, language is an issue. In North American manual therapy, the word "direct" refers to a direct stretch technique, and the word "indirect" describes a direction of ease technique. However, in Europe, the word "direct" refers to working directly on an affected organ or tissue, while the word "indirect" describes treating another structure to affect an organ or tissue. This book uses the European definitions.

An example of an Indirect Technique, which is treatment of one structure to affect another, could be treatment of the kidneys. There are muscles known as the psoas muscle that attach from the lower spine to the top of the leg. One stretches these muscles when doing a lunge stretch. Moving the legs activates the psoas muscles. This in turn can be used to release the kidneys, as these muscles move the spine away from the kidneys. This can be beneficial either where the structure is too difficult to contact and address directly (such as with the lungs), or where the structure is too painful to be treated directly.

## Motility Induction

Motility is a valuable method that may be used as a stand-alone treatment or after the release of a tissue. Motility is the intrinsic motion of each tissue. It is believed to allow fluid exchange, thereby releasing waste products and allowing nutrition to reach the structures. A person's Motility is around seven to eight cycles per minute and occurs in three dimensions. In VM this rhythm can be assessed, and should be symmetrical from side to side and have a smooth, regular quality. If it doesn't, Induction can be used, which involves following and encouraging the rhythm into its easiest and smoothest motions. (See Figure 6.6.) This in turn allows Motility to become more full and even. It brings the organ into equilibrium. At this point the practitioner will follow the rhythmic motion for a few cycles to ensure the nervous system has been reeducated to the proper, healthy, full, rhythmic motion the organ should have. This technique may be used after Mobility treatment, but is also effective where Mobility techniques are contraindicated or might be too invasive. Such can be the case in the treatment of babies, pregnant women, post-surgery cases, cases of acute bowel flare up, and the like. It is also used as the treatment of choice where the Listening takes a practitioner within the functional parts of an organ itself.

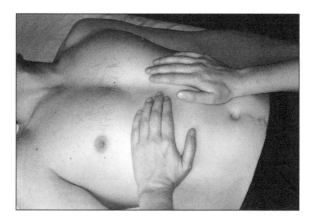

Figure 6.6. Motility balance technique on liver and stomach

## Other Treatments

A fuller discussion of emotions, blood vessels, and nerves is included later, along with the treatment techniques relevant to each of these specific components.

## Effects of Treatment

The effects of treatment vary, depending on the patient and on the techniques used. During the treatment session the practitioner will be looking for certain changes in the body that indicate the tissues are releasing.

The patient may also be aware of some of these changes. These include the following:

1. A tissue change, such as tissue softening (including reduced muscular tone or tissue tension), tissue lengthening, or improved tissue movement, which includes a renewed slide and glide between organs.

2. Increased fluid flow. This may be noticed by a change in swelling or pulse.

3. Increased energy flow. Often a greater feeling of vitality is apparent in an area that has just been treated.

4. Heat or temperature change. This can be a local effect or a more general effect on the body. It may also be seen by color changes in the skin, usually due to improved circulation or release of energy from the restricted tissues.

5. Breathing. Often, as tissues release it will allow the breathing to become fuller and less labored. This is a good sign of release in the body.

6. Emotional change. Sometimes as an area is released, one that has possibly had an emotional component, the patient may experience the edge of that emotion. It is not unusual for someone to be overcome with a feeling, such as sadness, anger, or a deep tranquility as the tissues change. In some instances a person may find a tear run down his or her face as the practitioner is treating a restricted organ.

7. Improved rhythm. There are various rhythms the practitioner monitors in the body—including the Motility of organs, the arterial pulse, the breathing, or the craniosacral rhythm. They will be looking for better symmetry and more balance in these rhythms as the tissues change.

8. Autonomic nervous system activity. This includes sudden muscular twitches or rapid eye movements. These are indications for the practitioner that the nervous system functioning is changing.

## After Treatment

Treatment may result in changes in many areas: posture, the ability to move, circulation in the body, the function of nerves, muscular tone or spasms, hormonal and chemical states, immunity, and emotions. A person may feel more energetic and flexible, and have a greater sense of well-being. On the other hand, sometimes after treatment the patient may feel tired, achy, stiff, or even appear to have more pain or new symptoms. The body has probably moved in new ways during the session or following it. Like any new type of exercise, VM uses muscles and the body in ways that may not have been done in a long time. It can take a few days to get used to this changed function.

It is not unusual for the released areas to have ripple effects into the surrounding tissues and lead to changed sensations in various parts of the body. A patient may also notice sweatiness, fever, headaches, mild nausea, or changed urine smell after treatment due to detoxification reactions. These can be minimized by drinking adequate amounts of water after treatment.

Any or all of the aforementioned changes are possible, due to the interconnectedness of the whole body. It is quite normal for these effects to last several days after a treatment session.

Following treatment it is advisable to take it a little easier to give the body a chance to continue the adaptation and healing process. It is a good idea to make sure to drink enough fluids—3 to 4 pints (1.5 to 2.0 l) per day—not partake in extreme exercise, and get enough rest. One should create a space to allow the body to get the maximum benefits from a treatment session whenever possible.

## Low Back Pain and Indigestion
## Require a Range of Treatment Techniques

For clarification on how the various techniques are applied during a VM session, in the patient case below, the techniques have been italicized.

### *The Fiddle Player*

Isobel was a thirty-five-year-old professional fiddle player. She was suffering from back pain and indigestion. She had seen a chiropractor for her back pain, which improved with treatment but then recurred a few days later. She was desperate to resolve these problems, as they really affected her while she stood and played her fiddle in her ceilidh band (traditional Scottish music) all evening in a gig.

Using General Listening I was taken to her right triangular ligament, which attaches the liver to the diaphragm. Local Listening also revealed issues with her stomach. Inhibition confirmed the right triangular ligament was the priority at that moment in time.

Treatment started with Isobel sitting. I worked *directly* on her liver to lift it and initially started with a *direction of ease technique,* taking her liver to the right once it was lifted. There were few signs of release, so I then took her liver to the left to do a *direct stretch* to her right triangular ligament. There was a little release, but only a minimal amount. So I decided to use a *Recoil* technique to wake up the ligament and hopefully allow release. With Isobel lying on her left side I placed one hand on her liver and crossed the other hand over it to reach the area of her diaphragm. I made sure I had contacted the liver and taken up tension by *stacking* into 3 planes. Then at the start of her inhalation, I quickly removed my hands. When I went back to feel the area I could feel *heat,* and I noticed her *breathing had become a bit deeper,* which are both *signs of release.* When I retested the Mobility of her right triangular ligament there was a much greater ability for it to stretch *(tissue lengthening)* when her liver was taken toward her left side.

On reevaluation her liver was no longer showing as the primary area of restriction. Now her stomach was the main issue. With Isobel sitting I assessed the Mobility of her stomach. I found it restricted in movement from right to left, and from moving down toward her feet. I started to release the restrictions in the vertical direction. With Isobel sitting, I contacted her stomach below her left ribs and anchored it with my thumb. Then I got Isobel to put both her hands behind her neck and lifted her elbows up and slightly to her right using them as a *long lever* to help with the stretch. I felt a lot of *softening* under my thumb on her stomach and then felt the *tension reduce* on the stretch that was being created by lifting her arms. Her stomach also let out gurgle, indicating *increased fluid flow.*

On reassessment I found her stomach freer, although with still some restriction in a right-to-left direction. Local Listening revealed this to be her lesser omentum, a ligamentous connection from her liver to her stomach. Supporting her liver and finding the precise *line of tension* to her stomach allowed her stomach to regain its Mobility. Then I balanced the liver and stomach *Motility* with one another, using *Induction* to encourage them to become synchronous.

After two further, similar treatments, Isobel reported that she had just completed an entire weekend of playing. It had been a traditional music festival and even though she had eaten poorly, she did not suffer from back pain or indigestion. It seems that the organ restrictions were creating a tension in her back, which was why the chiropractic care helped but the pain kept returning.

7

# Organs Overview

In a book where, until now, I have consistently commented that VM focuses on treating the body as a whole, it may seem strange to break the body up into systems. However, the body is too complex to discuss solely as one unit. For that reason only, I will now discuss the body systems individually. Primarily, this chapter is a discussion of the many factors that are common to all internal organs.

Internal organs rely on their position in the body and having enough support, space, movement, and nerve and blood/fluid supply to allow them to function optimally. In cases of organ dysfunction these factors are almost always compromised.

## Mechanical Support System

### *Fascia*

Immediately surrounding the organ is a layer called fascia. Fascia is a fine, smooth, stretchy, sausage-skin-like layer that is responsible for both containing the organ and allowing its smooth movement against adjacent structures. Actually, fascia does not only cover organs, but rather surrounds almost all body tissues. There are many types of fascia, including some specialized ones that surround nerves, the brain, muscles, and joints. It is continuous, meaning that all fascia is connected, so a person could follow fascia from the big toe to any other point on the body without having to leave it. Fascia is also able to stretch so that the tissues are able to move inside it. For example, when an arm bends, the fascia around the biceps muscle has to stretch to allow the muscle contained within it to work. Ligaments, tendons, peritoneum, meninges, and nerve sheaths are all types of fascia, all with slightly different structures to allow their specialized functions.

Fascia is formed from three components. These are collagen, elastin, and ground substance. The quantities of each of these components can vary, and they determine the properties of each area of fascia. For example, the fascia directly surrounding an organ such as the stomach would have to be very stretchy. Elastin (like "elastic") is the stretchy component, so there is likely to be a large proportion of elastin in this area. Collagen is a much stronger fiber but not very stretchy. So, a tendon would be formed of a large proportion of collagen and relatively little elastin. Ground substance is the lubricating material, which supplies nutrients and removes waste products along with housing a nerve supply for the fascia.

Fascia can become affected in different ways, like being overstretched, torn, or exposed to air (which causes it to become stickier). Any of these can affect the fascia's functions, so it may lose its ability to stretch properly. When this happens an organ may not be able to expand fully and its function may be impaired. Alternatively, it may happen that the fascia is no longer as smooth, and therefore sticks to the nearby tissues and anchors the organ so it cannot glide against its neighbors. Or perhaps the fascia has lost some of its elasticity, which leads to the organ not being supported properly via its connecting ligaments. This lack of support or slight change in position of the organ leads to dysfunction.

Fascia appears to have a "memory" for its optimal shape. It knows where it was when it was functioning well and has the ability to return toward its optimum position. Once the tensions that have affected it are removed, the fascia will attempt to return to its original, most effective shape. The role of Visceral Manipulation is to assist fascial function, to allow it to regain its stretch, reduce any scarring or stickiness, redistribute fluids, allow optimum nerve function and circulation, to restore chemical balance and to reestablish the memory pattern of the fascia.

## Muscles

The muscular system helps support the organs. Poor abdominal muscle tone allows a person to "gain a belly." As many of the internal organs rely on abdominal tone to help keep them in place and allow them to function perfectly, a general loss of tone in the abdomen may cause some of the organs to function less effectively. Muscular problems can be due to a lack of exercise, but also sometimes due to poor nerve supply or circulation to the muscles. Very commonly, despite symptoms being in a muscle, the cause lies elsewhere in the body. The muscles in the back can sometimes go into adaptive shortening in response to a spasm in the organ that lies just in front of them. For example the psoas muscle (hip flexor muscle) responds in this way to tension in the duodenum (part of the small intestine).

## Bones

The bony skeletal system can affect the internal organs. It is common for joints to become restricted, and this affects a person's movement. This can result in reduced Mobility of the organs because of the tensions and pulls around them that come from the muscles and fascia that attach to the bones.

## Pressure Systems

There are pressure systems that help support our organs. For example, the chest normally has a negative pressure due to the amount of air in the lungs, which helps pull up the organs in the upper abdomen. If this were not the case the body would not be able to hold up the 3- to 4-pound (1.5 kg) weight of the liver. These pressure systems are affected by movement, and by bodily functions such as breathing, coughing, or bearing down. Each organ also has its own mini-pressure system, which allows the organs to occupy their full space and not collapse in on themselves. Due to the pressure systems of the body, if astronauts went out into space without space suits, they would explode before they suffocated because there is no air pressure in space.

### Nerve System

The nerve system will be discussed in much more detail in Chapter Fifteen; however, it is important to point out that muscle, blood vessel, and organ tone are dependent on a well-functioning nerve supply. Additionally, movement of the organs is governed by nerve supply—from the functions of the one hundred and twenty thousand heartbeats per day to the twenty-four thousand breaths per day to the activity of peristalsis in moving food through the digestive system.

### Fluid Balance

The fluid balance of the body is vital for organ function; this will be discussed in Chapter Eleven. Put simply, fluid balance is crucial for each individual cell, the blood supply, and fluid lubrication of an organ as well as its surroundings. Where there is fluid congestion (known as edema) or dehydration, the function of the tissues quickly becomes impaired.

### Chemical Balance

Chemical balance, both through hormones and the balances of acidity or alkalinity in the body, affects how the tissues function. For example, in pregnancy, hormonal balance changes, allowing the tissues to have more elasticity to accommodate the growing baby and the extra movement required for delivery.

## Causes of Organ Dysfunction

Visceral Manipulation addresses the organs structurally by considering how they are able to move and function within and in relation to the tissues surrounding them. There are lots of factors that can lead to restrictions of these surrounding tissues, and these restrictions can have a significant effect on an organ's ability to move and function. The factor leading to dysfunction does not have to be of recent origin. It is possible that a past event has led to a change in the tissue—perhaps through the formation of scar tissue, or by allowing air into a liquid space and thus changing the stickiness of the liquid and the ability of tissues to slide against each other. Or an event can lead to a change in the nature of the tissue, either making it harder or looser. This can make it more or less supportive, or restrict the organs and tissues to which it relates. With tissue changes, perhaps stemming from an earlier event or from aging, the body loses its ability to compensate and a person starts to suffer symptoms.

Following are the most common factors that can affect the organs:

**Trauma.** The trauma can be directly on the organ, or it can result from damage to one of the tissues surrounding an organ. It can come from a neighboring organ, the skeletal system, or be transmitted via pressure changes elsewhere in the body. These could be from an accident or blow to the body. For example, in some car accidents there may be no direct trauma to the body, but the deceleration forces are so high that they cause pressure changes and damage to the body tissues. (See Figure 7.1.) Trauma can also be caused by temperature changes—perhaps burns or radiation or chemical trauma such as acid burns or poisoning.

**Surgery.** Any surgery creates adhesions. Letting air into the tissues where air would not usually be changes the stickiness of the fluids. This causes fascia and other tissues to stick together, creating adhesions.

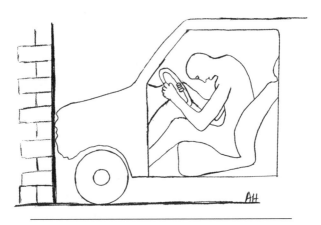

Figure 7.1. The effects of a car accident on a body

**Scars.** Scars are areas where tissues have healed. However, as most people know from personal experience, scars never quite return to a perfect state. Usually a scar leaves a raised area or mark on the body. (See Figure 7.2.) In some cases, some of the fine layers in the body may have stuck together. If so, they can prevent the tissues from moving as they should and lead to problems. Such problems can surface years later, as scar tissues change and tighten over time.

**Infection.** When there is an infection, the body attempts to wall it off from the surrounding tissues. The result, once the infection has passed,

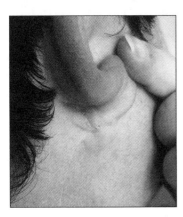

Figure 7.2. The tension caused by a scar

can be a dry, tethered area. This will pull the surrounding tissue toward it and create a tension in the body. Visceral Manipulation does not deal with the acute phase of an infection, but rather with the chronic consequences of the mechanical restrictions it can leave behind.

**Postural habits.** If someone has a round-shouldered posture, the organs in the front of the body become a little compressed. As a result, the lungs are not able to expand fully and thereby become compromised. (See Figure 7.3.) For this reason, one of the factors a VM practitioner considers on initial examination is the patient's posture.

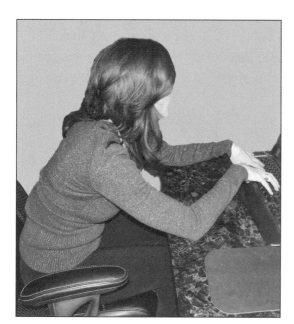

Figure 7.3. The effects of slouching on the body

**Gravity.** Gravity is a continuous force, with all human beings throughout their lives unless, of course, they decide to become astronauts. However, gravity means that with changes in posture the organs may experience pressures that affect them negatively and lead to further compensations in the body.

**Chemical.** Chemical factors include diet, fluid intake, allergies, drugs, vaccinations, or medications a person uses. These can affect the organs and lead to structural changes and restrictions. For example, having an allergy may lead to tissue inflammation.

**Inflammation.** This causes the tissues to swell, which will impact their function and the function of the other tissues around them. Inflammation can lead to stagnation in the lymphatic system (part of the immune system). This in turn can lead to further congestion and restriction in the tissues, both physically and chemically.

**Emotional state.** Every high emotional state affects an organ. (For more information on this, see the chapter on emotions, Chapter Sixteen.) Additionally, emotional states will affect the tissues surrounding an organ. Have you noticed that people tend to clench their muscles when they feel stressed?

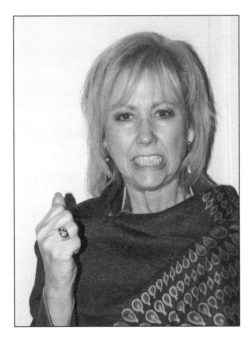

Figure 7.4. The tension created by stress in the body

**Muscle tone and spasm.** Spasm can either be of the muscle of the organ itself (for example, the digestive tubes have muscle in their walls to push the food along) or of the muscles surrounding the organs (for example, abdominal muscle tone). The tone may be increased or decreased, depending on the issue.

**Nerves and circulation.** The nerve and circulatory function is paramount to organ function. There can be tensions in blood vessels that become translated to an organ, or the supply to an organ itself may be altered. This is commonly caused by one of the factors listed above. For more details, please see the chapters on circulation and nerve manipulation, Chapters Eleven and Fifteen.

Where there is dysfunction of one organ or its surrounding tissues, it must be remembered that this will often affect other organs, via one of the following:

- fascial connections
- direct pressure onto a neighboring organ
- its blood or nerve supplies, or
- a lesional chain (see Chapter Four).

Although I will now discuss each system individually, the separation is purely academic. For example, in cases of a tension in the stomach (which belongs to the digestive system) it is not uncommon to find it affects the lungs (the respiratory system) and also the kidney (the waterworks), due to its geographical location in the body.

Visceral Manipulation addresses all the components of optimum organ functioning, from the emotions to the blood and nerve supply to the organ's position in the body. Other factors that may require advice are lifestyle, environmental, and chemical factors. For these reasons, a practitioner might make nutrition- or exercise-related recommendations, or suggest a visit to a specialist to help address these issues.

### Menstrual Pain and Constipation Resolve Simultaneously

A twenty-five-year-old woman named Leigh came to see me complaining of menstruation pain. She also reported that she tended to be constipated, often going several days between her bowel movements. She had lower abdominal pain and low back pain. This all seemed to have started after she had suffered from an infection.

General Listening took me to her pelvis. Local Listening her uterosacral ligament seemed to be the primary issue. This ligament runs back from the uterus to the sacrum (tailbone area); between the uterus and sacrum lies the rectum. With Leigh lying on her back, I placed one hand on her belly and one on her sacrum. I did a direction of ease release. This created a softening of the whole area, and the tension in her lower pelvic tissues greatly reduced. I then balanced Motility of her rectum and uterus.

When I saw her a month later, she reported her menstrual pain had significantly decreased, and she was much less constipated. She also had less back and abdominal pain. After three more sessions, at monthly intervals, she was satisfied with the outcome, having daily bowel movements and no low back pain. This shows how neighboring organs that belong to different organ systems can be affected by the same restriction due to their proximity.

8

# Digestive System

D igestion is something that is vital for survival. While people can go for a few weeks without food, the digestive system also takes fluids into human bodies, and survival is quickly threatened if they are stopped. Given that the average person in the West eats 55 tons (50 tonnes) of food, and drinks 11,000 gallons (50,000 l) of liquid during his or her life, this really is a remarkable processing system. (See Figure 8.1.) The digestive system is basically composed of a tube that runs from the mouth to the anus. It interacts with other organs, such as the liver, gallbladder, and pancreas. The tube itself is actually about 30 feet (9 m) long, but is folded and gathered in such a way it fits into our on average 2- to 3-foot-long (60 to 90 cm) torso.

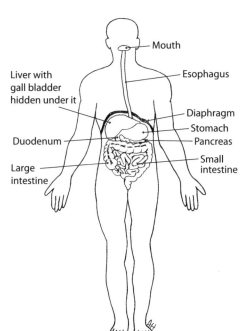

Mouth

Liver with gall bladder hidden under it

Esophagus

Diaphragm

Stomach

Pancreas

Duodenum

Small intestine

Large intestine

Figure 8.1. The digestive system

77

It is remarkable how clever the body is at supporting this tube, and at preventing kinks or twists from occurring. It is not surprising that at some time most people experience digestive discomfort or dysfunction. After someone eats an abnormally large meal or eats while sitting in a poor posture, the tube and its supports are tested to their limits. It is through treating the tube, its supports, its surrounding tissues, the junction points in the tube, and its related organs that it is possible for a VM practitioner to enhance someone's digestive function.

To help clarify the way the system works, I would liken digestion to the process a washing machine goes through as it breaks down dirt during its various cycles. I am not intimating that these cycles are the same, only using the comparison to illustrate the processes involved. Digestion and the washing machine rely on similar methods to process and breakdown substances. A washing machine uses physical agitation to loosen dirt, fluid to soften it, and detergent chemicals to complete the breakdown. Likewise, the digestive system uses mechanical breakdown, fluids, and chemicals (known as enzymes) to help process food. (See Figure 8.2)

The food a person eats is not in a useable form for the body. Physical breakdown starts at the point of entry, in the mouth. Here the teeth start the process, while the salivary glands add the first dose of fluid and chemicals. When food is swollowed it passes down the esophagus, a fairly straight and expandable part of the tube, to the stomach. It takes food seven seconds to pass down the average adult's 1-foot-long (25 cm) and 1-inch (2.5 cm) diameter esophagus. The esophagus is a highly muscular tube, which pushes the food toward the stomach. It is so strong that even if people eat food standing on their heads, the food will still end up in the stomach.

The stomach is a widened part of the tube that provides both mechanical and chemical breakdown. This could be likened to the main wash cycle in the washing machine, where there is mechanical agitation as the contents are soaked and detergent is added. The stomach has very muscular walls so, like the washing machine, it can start to agitate the food and break it into smaller parts while soaking it in acidic liquid. From the stomach, the food passes gradually into a long journey through various tubes, known as the intestines. In the first part of the intestines, the muscular-walled duodenum, further, more vigorous mechanical breakdown occurs, along with the addition of various enzymes (chemicals) that digest all the different food substances.

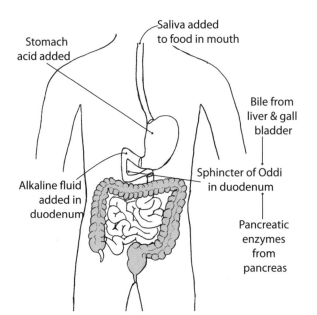

Figure 8.2. Fluids added to the digestive tract

Specialized enzymes are produced and stored by the digestive organs—the liver, gallbladder, and pancreas. This is like adding specific stain removers to your wash cycle. The liver and gallbladder work together for fat digestion. The liver produces a substance known as bile. Bile is a fat digester that is rather like dishwashing liquid and is even greenish in color. The production of bile is continuous, but it is not necessarily required at all times. If bile is not required, it goes up the cystic duct and is stored and concentrated in the gallbladder. When bile is required because a person has eaten a fatty meal, some bile is sent from the gallbladder and some freshly made bile comes from the liver. This is sent to the duodenum (a part of the small intestine) via the common bile duct. The pancreas also feeds into the duodenum at this point; the pancreas produces pancreatic enzymes, which are like extra detergent to further help the chemical breakdown of food.

The structure of the walls of the intestine changes as the food passes out of the duodenum and into the rest of the small intestines. Here the walls are much thinner and have an excellent blood supply. This is because this area is where the digested food is absorbed. This section is 21 feet (6.5 m) of coiled tubing, creating a very large surface area of 656 square feet (200 sq m) to allow for maximum absorption in minimum time. The nutrients are filtered out through the walls of the small intestine into the blood and are then carried by the blood off to the liver to be sorted, filtered, and distributed around the body.

Once absorption has occurred, the remains of the food pass into the large intestine (also known as colon). This is like the drainage cycle of the wash. Here the waste products are dehydrated and any final nutrients removed. The waste products are packaged up ready for passing via the rectum and anus when a person gets the call of nature. Constipation can result when too much water is absorbed in the large intestine and the waste matter becomes too dry.

Another important element of the system is a series of muscular rings that are found in the digestive tract. These act like valves that slow down or control the passage of substances from one stage to the next. These are known as sphincters; a more detailed description is below.

Finally, the fascia of the abdomen known as the peritoneum deserves a special mention. This is formed of two layers. An outer layer, known as the parietal peritoneum, lines the abdominal cavity. It has a good nerve supply and forms a bag around many of the digestive organs. It also has a reflex response and absorbs shock. In places, the organs pass through this layer. The internal layer, known as the visceral peritoneum, serves as fascia around many organs (the stomach and liver, for example) but acts as ligaments in some areas, for example, for suspending parts of the intestines. The peritoneum produces fluid that allows it and the organs it contains to glide across one another. If this fluid comes into contact with air (following surgery, for example) it can become stickier and lead to the formation of adhesions. Additionally, inflammation or trauma may affect the peritoneum. The peritoneum needs to be able to expand to allow the digestive system to function properly. It has a number of blood vessels and nerves that run through it that can also be affected by any tensions it has. It can contract or spasm. Also, if there is a restriction of the peritoneum, it can lead to other problems anywhere around the abdominal area. There are techniques in VM used to help free up the peritoneum and allow it to release to continue its functions and not place a strain on its surrounding tissues. Treatment usually involves the practitioner helping the peritoneum to regain its shear and glide, both with itself and in relation to the organs it contacts. This may be done with the patient in a lying position or on all fours, depending on the exact location of the restriction. (See Figure 8.3.) The peritoneum also has Motility, and in VM it is often balanced to allow better function of the abdominal tissues.

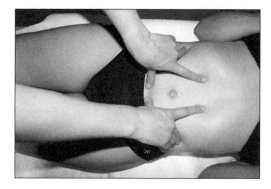

Figure 8.3. Peritoneum release

In other areas peritoneum that joins two organs together is known as omentum. It is a continuation of exactly the same structure, just with a different name, rather like a road that has several names along its route. There are two omenta—the lesser joins the liver to the stomach and duodenum, while the greater hangs underneath the stomach and is attached very loosely to the colon. The greater omentum is a fatty apron with a good blood and nerve supply that not only acts as a support in the abdominal cavity, but also has roles in the immune system and provides insulation and shock absorption through its fat content. If there is a restriction of the greater omentum it can cause a symptom of a "stitch," often felt after exercise or running. Treatment techniques may be done with the patient in a sitting, lying, or all-fours position, and involve freeing up the greater omentum in relation to the organs it covers.

## Further Details on Each Part of the Digestive System

### Stomach

As described above, the stomach has muscular walls and secretes acid and enzymes, allowing it to start the food breakdown process both mechanically and chemically. It is the widest part of the digestive tube and can contain three and 0.2 pints (1.5 l) of food and fluids. Every day it secretes 2 to 4 pints (1 to 2 l) of acid that is strong enough to dissolve razor blades. Fortunately, the cells in the stomach lining renew so quickly that the acids don't have time to dissolve it. People have a new lining for their stomachs every three days. Food is usually in the stomach for up to three hours after a meal, depending on what was eaten—it is slower for bodies to break down meat and fat than vegetables and carbohydrates. Due to the stomach's mechanical functions, stomach tone is very important.

The stomach is located on the left side of the body, toward the front. (See Figure 8.4.) The top part of it is covered by ribs. It is about 5 inches (12 cm) wide, 1.25 to 2.5 inches (3 to 6 cm) thick, and on average 10 inches (25 cm) long—although it is very common for the stomach to hang down below the level of the navel, especially after a meal. It is a hollow organ, meaning there is a space inside it. It is like a bag that holds and processes food, with an entrance at the top and exit at the bottom.

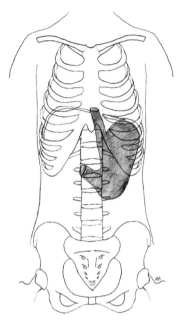

Figure 8.4. Stomach location

The stomach is supported by ligaments. These ligaments run at the top to the diaphragm, from the left side to the spleen and large intestine, and from the right side to the duodenum and liver. The stomach sits beside the pancreas, spleen, left kidney, and adrenal gland, the small and large intestines, and in some cases, the bladder if it has become lengthened. Additionally, the stomach can be influenced by the heart and lungs, which sit just above the diaphragm, on top of the stomach. From the stomach, the greater omentum hangs down and loops back onto the intestines. Through the greater omentum, the stomach can become aggravated by almost any abdominal organ, as the greater omentum covers over the whole front of the abdominal area.

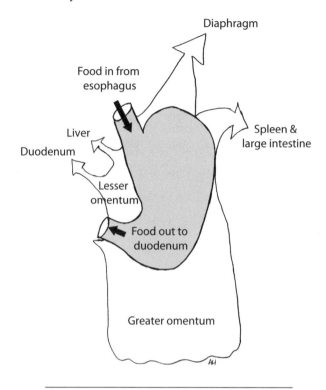

Figure 8.5. Stomach relations and attachments

Treatment of the stomach may be done with the patient sitting or lying down. As the lower part of the stomach is easily palpable at the front of the abdomen, practitioners may contact it there. For some techniques they may work through the ribs to reach the upper part of the stomach or perhaps to reach another organ that is restricted against the stomach, such as the liver. The aim of treatment is to ensure that the stomach is able to move and has the ability to slide and glide against the tissues surrounding it in three dimensions. This is achieved by treating its ligaments and relationships to surrounding organs. Additionally, the stomach needs to be able to move within itself to create the mechanical action to break down food, so part of treatment may be to encourage this motion. (See Figure 8.6.) It is likely the practitioner will address stomach Motility and sphincters (see below) as part of the treatment on a patient's stomach.

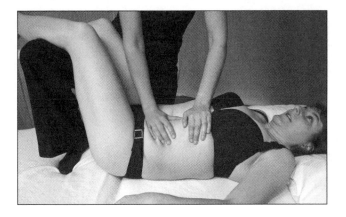

Figure 8.6. Mobility treatment of the stomach

Possible causes of stomach issues:

- Poor abdominal muscle tone
- Poor posture
- Surgery (abdominal)
- Endometriosis and sexually transmitted diseases
- Inflammation
- Scars
- Reduced lymphatic function
- Pregnancy and childbirth
- Allergies
- Chemicals
- Medication
- Trauma

Symptoms of stomach issues that may improve with VM:

- Hiatus hernias or pain increased over lower ribs with breathing
- Stomach ptosis, in which the stomach has become elongated and lowered

- Stomach ulcers
- Left-sided headaches
- Pain over stomach area, and avoidance of wearing tight clothes or belts
- Left shoulder pain
- Left-sided neck pain and restriction
- Mid-back pain and restriction
- Left low back pain
- Left sinus problems
- Short in-breaths
- Slow digestion
- Tiredness
- Excessive belching
- Throwing up or reflux
- Anemia

## *Child's Sickness Ends with Visceral Manipulation*

Angus, who was sixteen months old and had beautiful curly blond hair when he first came to see me, was vomiting up any solid food he was given. His mother had resorted to liquifying all of his food. She told me he was a very "sickly" baby and was developmentally slow, only recently being able to crawl.

When I looked at Angus I noted he was pale. With General Listening I was taken to the tissues in his chest area. With Local Listening I identified it as his esophagus, the pipe that links his mouth to his stomach. His stomach also was not able to move downward properly on Mobility testing, and his whole chest felt congested.

By engaging his chest and food pipe (esophagus), I was able to get his tissues to release. I then used a direction of ease technique that allowed his stomach to regain its freedom to descend easily. With Induction normal, Motility was restored. I suggested to his mother that she try giving him semisolid food.

At the next appointment, two weeks later, his mother reported with delight that Angus had only been sick twice and that he had started eating foods with soft lumps, such as soup. His color was better, and he looked much more alert. Following another two treatments Angus was able to eat most foods, although his mother did report that certain things like toast still sometimes posed a problem. He had also started crawling and was pulling himself up to standing, and generally seemed to be thriving.

Digestive issues can not only prove upsetting for the child and parent, but also affect development as the child struggles to have enough energy and nutrition. Visceral Manipulation often can locate and resolve these issues completely.

### Duodenum

Duodenum (part of the small intestine) means "two plus ten" in Latin, referring to its length as measured in finger sections. It is about 10 inches (25 cm) long, but is only about the thickness of your thumb. It is behind the layer called the peritoneum, which is the lining of the abdominal cavity. It lies toward the back of the abdominal cavity, close to the spine. The duodenum connects to the lower end of the stomach and then forms a C-shaped curve in the abdominal cavity before joining with the rest of the small intestines just above and to left of the navel. (See Figure 8.7.) It also has connections to the gallbladder and pancreas via the ducts that join the duodenum from those organs at the Sphincter of Oddi.

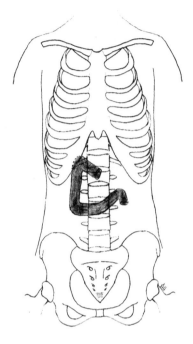

Figure 8.7. Duodenum location

The duodenum is in very close relationship with almost all the abdominal organs, with tissue associations to all the other digestive organs along with the abdominal aorta, the kidneys, and the ureter. (See Figure 8.8.) It has ligaments that attach it to the diaphragm and the spine. It crosses in front of the spine at the top of the lumbar area (low back), and when dysfunctional, the duodenum can mimic psoas muscle pain as it causes the psoas to shorten. At the top it is fed into by the stomach, and then the food passes into the rest of the small intestines once the duodenum has completed its mechanical and chemical breakdown of the food. As it is in contact with so many other organs, it can be influenced by a wide range of abdominal tensions and can be an important area in treatment.

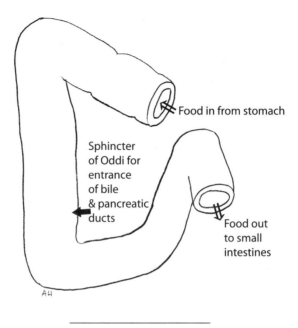

Sphincter
of Oddi for
entrance
of bile
& pancreatic
ducts

Food in from stomach

Food out
to small
intestines

Figure 8.8. The duodenum

As it lies so deep in the abdominal cavity, treatment will usually either be with the patient in a sitting position, lying on his or her back with knees bent, or lying on the right side. Treatment will focus on aiding the elongation of the tubes of the duodenum and its ligamentous attachments. Tubes respond very well to being elongated, and as the tube of the duodenum is so folded, this often needs to be done in various directions. A practitioner may use long levers, such as moving the trunk to encourage release of these tubes and ligaments. (See Figure 8.9.) Additionally, treatment may include balancing the duodenum with the spine, as it has connections to the spine through both its proximity and a ligament (called the ligament of Trietz). Motility will often be assessed and may be balanced with another organ, such as the stomach, depending on a person's particular case.

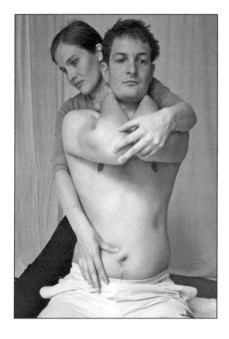

Figure 8.9. Duodenum
direct stretch

Possible causes of Duodenum issues:

- Mechanical injury—for example, by a seatbelt in a car accident
- Overproduction of acid or other chemical stress leading to spasms
- After surgery, commonly of the gallbladder
- Duodenal ulcers
- A dysfunctional pyloric sphincter allowing acid in from the stomach (see below)
- Emotional overflow of the mind
- Anxiousness
- Long-term social or professional frustration

Symptoms of duodenum issues that may improve with VM:

- Lower back pain, especially on the right
- Mid-back pain, which can mimic psoas pain

- Right-sided central abdominal pain
- Duodenal ulcers
- Pain from 2 a.m. to 4 a.m.
- Pain one and a half to three hours after eating
- Pain before breakfast relieved by food but not sugar

## Small Intestine

The small intestine (referring to the jejunoileum in this case) is one of the most remarkable pieces of engineering in the body. Some 22 feet (6.5 m) of tubing is folded and held in place, generally without getting tangled or restricted. One only has to think of how often the U-bend under the sink becomes blocked and then consider that there are fifteen or sixteen such U-bends in the small intestines—quite a plumbing job! (See Figure 8.10.) The intestines are attached to the back of the abdominal cavity just in front of the spine by a large ligament called the mesentery, which looks a bit like a big bunch of lettuce that has the tubing attached at the end of its leaves. The freedom of this large attachment is important to allow the full flow of blood and nerve supply that is fed to the small intestines through the lettuce-like mesentery. The function of the small intestines is absorption of nutrients; over their length, ninety percent of a person's digestive absorption occurs.

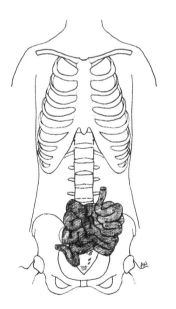

Figure 8.10. Small intestine location

As the small intestine is so expansive, it tends to interact with almost every abdominal and pelvic organ, the front abdominal wall, and the main blood vessels that take blood to and from the legs, known as the aorta and inferior vena cava, respectively. However, the most common sites of restrictions are the mesentery and the loops of the small intestine. When the small intestine is being treated, the patient will either will be lying on the back or the side. The practitioner may be feeling deeper into the abdomen to reach the mesentery and its root, or may be closer to the front surface treating some of the loops in the tubing. The aim will be to allow greater slide and glide between the structures. Often the practitioner will then finish up with Motility of the whole small intestine. (See Figure 8.11.)

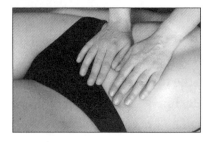

Figure 8.11. Small intestine Motility

Possible causes of small intestine issues:

- Fibrosis or adhesions
- Intestinal spasms
- Constipation or diarrhea
- Any surgical opening of the abdomen
- Trauma
- Stress or tension
- Allergies or reactions to food
- Infections affecting the digestive tract
- Psoas muscles spasm
- Circulatory restrictions to the small intestines

Symptoms of small intestine issues that may improve with VM:

- Poor digestion
- Low energy
- Food sensitivities
- Deep bone ache (due to calcium deficiency)
- Low back pain or restriction
- Left sided sciatica
- Joint pain in the legs
- Poor circulation
- Weakness in legs or cold or itchy feet
- Restless leg syndrome
- Does not want to wear tight clothing or belts
- Insomnia
- Tiredness, especially on waking but improving in the middle of the day
- Hernias
- Does not digest salads well, especially cucumbers, tomatoes, and cabbage

### *Abdominal Bloating and Indigestion Following a Hysterectomy and Bladder Lift*

Moira was referred to me by another chiropractor after her general health had improved through treatment but her ongoing digestive problems had not changed. When I first met Moira she reported that she regularly felt bloated after eating. She felt like she could not digest her meals properly and so had to eat only a little at a time. She told me that she had been to see her doctor, who had told her she had irritable bowel syndrome. She also explained that she could not drink alcohol as that further exacerbated her problems. She did miss this, as she enjoyed a glass of wine with her husband at dinner, especially now as they were both retired. Moira told me she'd had a hysterectomy eight years previously, and a bladder lift and bowel repair following that.

When I did General Listening on Moira I was pulled to her right lower abdomen, close to the midline of her body. I felt this area and found that it felt firmer than what would normally be expected. Using Local Listening, there was a pull up to the lower end of the root of her mesentery. Moira reported it all felt tender when I touched the area. Her small intestine had a sluggish Motility and was held on Expir, which would indicate a restriction in the flow of fluids relating to the small intestine. The firmer area in her lower abdomen appeared to have resulted from adhesions following her surgeries.

I softly engaged the tissues in the lower abdomen, which encouraged them to release. Gradually, as they freed up, with a significant discharge of heat, there was less of a pull to the root of the mesentery and peritoneum. I went on to release each side of the root of the mesentery and then balanced Motility using Induction for the whole of the small intestine.

The next time I saw Moira, a few weeks later, she told me that she had suffered significantly less bloating and indigestion except for on the day following treatment, when it had been particularly bad. During this second session I continued treating her adhesions and the small intestine. From that point on she had no further bloating or indigestion on a regular basis. During her Mediterranean cruise holiday, which she went on the week after treatment, she even started to drink a little wine again without any symptoms.

---

### Large Intestine and Rectum

The large intestine (also known as the colon) connects to the lower end of the small intestine at the cecum. It runs from the lower right corner of the abdominal cavity up the right side of the abdomen (ascending colon), across the body (transverse colon) and then down the left side of the abdomen (descending colon) to the sigmoid colon and then connects to the rectum. (See Figures 8.12 and 8.13.). The large intestine is considerably wider than the small intestine. It starts as 3 inches (7 to 8 cm) wide but narrows down to 1 inch (3 cm) by the time it reaches the rectum. Due to its length and layout it interacts with all the other abdominal and pelvic organs, along with the front and back abdominal walls and the diaphragm.

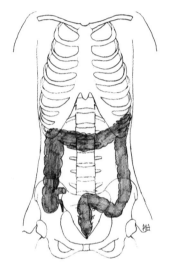

Figure 8.12. Large intestine location

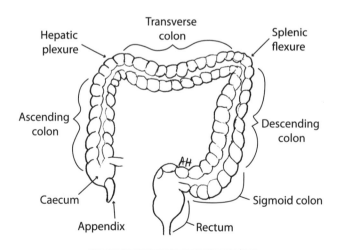

Figure 8.13. The large intestine

The rectum forms the end of the road for the unused parts of all meals. It is the final section of the digestive tube leading to the anus. It is 8 inches (20 cm) long, curved, and lies just in front of the tailbone. At the lower end of the rectum is the anus, which is a sphincter (valve-like function) that can tighten or release to allow bowel movements.

The large intestine is suspended and attached throughout its length by various folds of peritoneum, but generally loosely enough that it can move and expand with the changing volume of its contents. For this reason, when there is any abdominal or pelvic tension the large intestine is likely to be addressed. Likewise, the large intestine can affect any other abdominal or pelvic organ, or the pressure systems of the body, through constipation or diarrhea and the forces these place on the surrounding tissues and ligaments. Additionally, the hard frame (bony structures), especially in the pelvic area, may be affected by, or have an affect on the function of the large intestines or the rectum. This means that issues involving the large intestines may underlie chronic back pain or sacro-iliac problems.

When treating the large intestine and rectum, the basic principle used in VM is to help the tube to elongate, free up the corners in the tube, and make sure that the tube has its normal amount of slide and glide in relation to the organs and ligaments surrounding it. Due to the length of the large intestine and to the different attachments and locations it occupies over its course, the practitioner may ask the patient to sit, or lie on either side or on his or her back, depending on the exact restrictions. (See Figure 8.14.) The practitioner may also ask the patient to help by moving the legs or body in a particular way to increase the elongation of the tissues when during the application of Direct Techniques. The practitioner will also balance the Motility of the large intestine. In some instances the most effective treatment for the rectum may be to work internally to fully resolve the issue, and some VM practitioners may be trained to do this internal treatment.

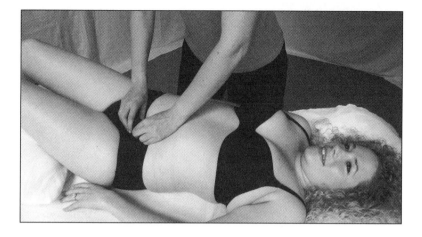

Figure 8.14. Treatment of the sigmoid colon

Possible causes of large intestine issues:

- Restrictions of the sacroiliac joints
- Issues of the urogenital organs or kidneys
- Digestive dysfunction, such as diarrhea or constipation
- Crohn's disease or ulcerative colitis
- Surgical opening of the abdomen
- Appendicitis
- Stress or tension

Symptoms of large intestine or rectum issues that may improve with VM:

- Low back or pelvic pain, either acute or chronic
- Sacroiliac problems
- Abdominal pain
- Sciatica
- Varicose veins
- Joint pain of the lower limbs

- Stinging eyes
- Waking up at night
- Problems with eating late at night
- "Dull cloud" feeling mentally
- Right shoulder pain
- Colitis, bowel inflammation, or hemorrhoids
- Wind (flatulence)
- Diarrhea or constipation

### *Abdominal Pain without Diagnosis*

William's mother was a patient of mine when I lived and worked in the south of England, before I moved back to my native Scotland. I was most surprised when one day a year or so after I had moved she called my clinic to talk about her son. He had been suffering severe abdominal pains to the point he had been taken into Great Ormond Street Hospital in London (a world-renowned children's hospital), and they put him on a drip to "settle his digestive system." They provided no further treatment other than having found he had an allergy to dairy. Eventually they reintroduced him to food and sent him home. At the age of ten, he appeared unwell and had recurrent episodes of abdominal pain.

William's mother decided to fly up to Scotland with him to see me. General and Local Listening took me to his cecum, at the upper end of his large intestine, and the area of the ileocaecal valve. I started by freeing up this area, as it felt incredibly restricted. William often had times of constipation, which is commonly caused by a restriction of the cecum. I used both direction of ease and direct stretch techniques to free it up. Until this point there was very little Motility of his cecum. The next thing I checked was the functioning of the sphincters (see below for full discussion of them). In his case, the ileocaecal valve was frozen. I used a Recoil technique and then Induction to encourage it to return to a functional state. Once it freed up it also restored functional Motility of another sphincter, which had been dysfunctional secondary to the ileocaecal valve.

Because he lived so far away, I did not see William for a couple of months. When I saw him again his mother reported he had greatly improved, and was now eating more and gaining some of the weight he had lost. He still had occasional episodes, but much less severe than previously.

On evaluation I found his large intestine had reasonable Motility and much improved Mobility. My treatment was to free up the remaining restrictions. My suspicion in this case was that the allergy to dairy was causing an inflammatory response, which in turn caused restrictions of his digestive system. However, once the dairy was removed from his diet he did not fully recover until the restrictions were also released and his digestive system had the freedom to commence normal functioning.

One of the great joys I have when using VM is being able to find answers for people who have become frustrated by their health. VM looks at different aspects that do not necessarily show up on conventional tests and are often not considered elsewhere. In my clinic I see a large proportion of chronic patients, that is, people who have had their condition for a long time and often come to me as a last resort. It gives me great happiness and feeds my enthusiasm for VM on a daily basis to hear stories of how these people have been helped by it.

*Liver*

As mentioned above, the liver has several roles in digestion—producing bile, as well as storing, filtering, and distributing nutrients to the body. It also is involved in balancing hormonal levels, producing heat, and managing and detoxifying the blood. In total, there are more than five hundred functions the liver performs. It is a large and heavy organ, weighing around 3 to 4 pounds (1 to 1.5 kg). As much as 3.2 pints (1.5 l) of blood per minute pass through it, and it has a large network of blood vessels.

The liver is located on the right side of your body, mostly under the lower ribs. (See Figure 8.15.) It is triangular in shape. Width-wise, the liver runs about three quarters of the way across the body. At the left side is a thin corner, but at the right side its depth is nearly half the height of the rib cage. It is also thick in a front-to-back direction, filling more than half the depth of the body.

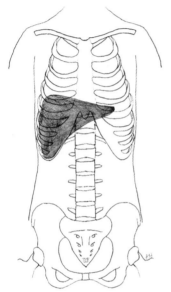

Figure 8.15. Liver location

The main movement (Mobility) restrictions of the liver usually occur because of either its relation to other organs or its ligament attachments, the latter which help to support the liver in place. The liver sits above the kidney, the gallbladder, the large intestine, the stomach, and the duodenum, and beneath the diaphragm, with the lungs and heart above it. The liver is attached via ligaments to the diaphragm, the front abdominal wall, the right kidney, the large intestine, the duodenum, the esophagus and the stomach. (See Figure 8.16.) Because of these attachments, dysfunction of any of the above organs can lead to issues for the liver, and vice versa. A restriction of an organ can lead to a loss of tissue independence, in this case making the liver unable to slide and glide with its neighboring organs and tissues. This can create significant aches, pains, and movement restrictions throughout the body. For example, to forward bend, the spine must move, but also the liver has to slide over the large intestine. If it does not, a person will be unable to touch his or her toes.

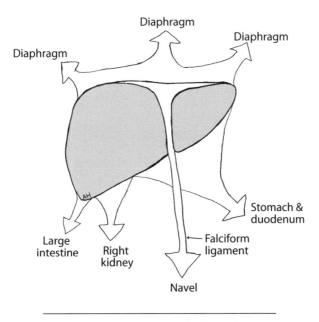

Figure 8.16. Liver relations and attachments

To reach the liver, the practitioner will have the patient either sitting in a slumped position or lying on the back or left side. It is possible for trained VM practitioners to directly feel the bottom edge of the liver up under the ribs, or they may work through the ribs to reach the liver, using slight compression to access the liver tissues. Treatment will be focused on allowing the liver to move freely in its anatomical environment; that is, in relation to its surrounding organs and ligaments. (See Figure 8.17.) Once the liver is moving well with its surrounding tissues, the practitioner will address its intrinsic motion (Motility) and perhaps balance it with other nearby organs.

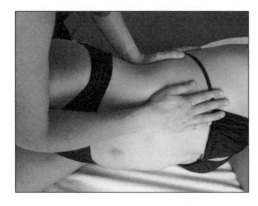

Figure 8.17. Liver Mobility

Possible causes of liver issues:

- Infection
- Trauma such as traffic accidents (as it is so large and relatively solid, shock waves from trauma often affect the liver)
- Strong emotions or depression
- Increased hormonal levels
- Medications
- Alcohol intake
- Poor diet
- Chest infections or a lot of coughing
- Issues of the right kidney
- Digestive problems

Symptoms of liver dysfunction that may improve with VM:

- Right-sided symptoms
- Right-sided headaches and scalp sensitivity
- Right-sided frozen shoulder
- Right shoulder pain or restriction
- Mid-neck restriction or pain
- Sciatica
- Restrictions of the mid-spinal region

- Chronic right sinusitis
- Acute sense of smell
- Photophobia (being very light sensitive)
- Night hyperthermia—feeling hot being unable to sleep at night
- Varicosities (e.g., varicose veins and hemorrhoids)
- Oily hair and dandruff
- Hypersensitive skin
- Tiredness
- Dull complexion
- Insomnia or sleep that brings no rest
- A decrease in fighting spirit

### Chronic Fatigue Syndrome and the Liver

A thirty-five-year-old Canadian gentleman named Kyle, who had moved to Scotland, came to see me about his chronic fatigue syndrome (CFS), which he had suffered with for at least ten years. Kyle reported that he felt tired and hypersensitive and had poor concentration and short-term memory. He had a general stiffness and achiness of the joints, and generally could not be bothered with anything. His theory was that he was suffering from various infections and heavy metal poisoning. Like many people with long-term health conditions, Kyle was very well-read and had researched possible causes on the Internet.

With General Listening I was taken to his right side, just below the ribs. I went on to do Manual Thermal Evaluation and Local Listening, which confirmed that it was a restriction affecting his liver. With Local Listening his liver felt pulled up to its top right corner. I Mobility tested his liver, and found it was harder to move from right to left and toward his navel. This indicated a restriction of his right triangular ligament, a ligament that attaches the right part of the liver to the diaphragm. Additionally, there was a pull into his circulatory system that went down toward his legs.

I started to treat the right triangular ligament of his liver. Gradually some Mobility started to return. Although the treatment was to stretch the ligament in one plane (two dimensionally), the effects mean that the liver regains its capacity to slide with the structures on all sides of it and so treatment has a three-dimensional effect.

The pull through Kyle's circulatory system seemed related to the tension his liver placed on the inferior vena cava, which is the large vessel that brings blood back to the heart from the lower half of the body. The liver sits directly in front of it and has a ligament that attaches around this vessel. When Kyle's liver finally freed up, the pull and tension into the circulatory system also reduced, and by his following appointment with me his lower limbs felt less congested.

Kyle reported that over this time he found he had more energy and had gradually felt his concentration and memory were improving. He also noted that his enthusiasm for life was increasing, as would fit with the emotional reactions of the liver. He found it was easier to use his legs and he was able to stand for a longer period of time without tiring, although he did still have some joint stiffness.

Chronic Fatigue Syndrome is not a straightforward condition, often only being diagnosed in lieu of any other clear diagnosis. It is often long term, has a complicated cause, and can be extremely debilitating. While the issues with Kyle's liver certainly played a large part in his condition, he is continuing with treatment to help his body regain more normal functioning. We are now treating other issues that were already in his body but were not as dominant as his liver issue.

---

### Gallbladder

The gallbladder has the purpose of storing and concentrating bile, which digests fats. It is not essential for life; I am sure we all know people who have had their gallbladders removed. However, its removal may mean that it is less easy for the person to digest fats, as the only bile being put into the duodenum following a fatty meal enters at the rate at which the liver makes it.

The gallbladder has a relatively simple structure—it is a small pouch that hangs under the liver and has one tube, known as the cystic duct, through which bile passes in and out of the gallbladder. (See Figure 8.18.) It is highly attached to the liver and only the very end of the gallbladder has any movement independent of the liver, hence it may be treated alongside your liver.

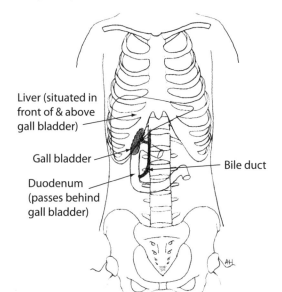

Figure 8.18. Gallbladder location

Ligaments from the gallbladder also attach to the duodenum (via the cystic duct in the hepatoduodenal ligament) and to the large intestine. The cystic duct runs into the common bile duct, which connects to the duodenum at the *sphincter of Oddi,* so the gallbladder, duodenum, and sphincter of Oddi can affect one another. (See Figure 8.19.) The sphincter of Oddi is a valve that controls the flow of fluids and allows them into but not out of the duodenum.

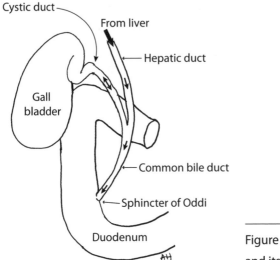

Figure 8.19. The gallbladder
and its ducts

The most common issue with the gallbladder relates to a blockage
of the tubes or sphincters it feeds into. These lead to a backpressure
into the gallbladder and may lead to stagnation, resulting in gallstones.
Alternatively, the bile may become thicker due to chemical changes that
lead to blockage of the gallbladder and its tubes. Many gallbladder problems and stones have no symptoms—it is estimated half the population
have gallbladder issues, and many people will never know about them.
Indeed there can be a huge number of stones in the gallbladder; a woman
from Berlin, Germany, had 3,110 gallstones taken out of her gallbladder. Gallstone issues may or may not be treatable with VM, depending
on their size and location. Even after gallbladder removal many people
still suffer symptoms, as the area of the gallbladder still holds tension
through surgical scarring. In these cases VM can be very beneficial in
helping to resolve post-surgical adhesions.

The gallbladder lies about halfway out to the right side of the body,
tucked under the lower ribs and under the liver. Usually release is done
with the patient sitting slumped forward a little. Due to the gallbladder's

close relationship with the liver, the liver may be treated first. Additionally, the practitioner will probably stretch out the tubing from the gallbladder to the duodenum and may ask the patient to lie on his or her back for that stage. The practitioner may also check the sphincter of Oddi to be sure bile drainage is optimal following treatment, and then balance the Motility of the gallbladder.

Possible causes of gallbladder issues:
- Superficial daily stress, such as stress of travelling
- Immediate bad news
- Increased hormonal levels (higher levels can increase risk of gallstones)
- Medications, especially for increased blood pressure
- Sphincter of Oddi dysfunction
- Very fatty diet

Symptoms of gallbladder issues that may improve with VM:
- Pain in right side of abdomen
- Pain in left shoulder blade or shoulder, due to left phrenic nerve, which supplies the gallbladder. (Developmentally, the gallbladder began on the left side of the body.)
- Restrictions between the shoulder blades on the right
- Neck pain and headaches
- Breathing changes—usually shallower breathing, as breathing deeper puts pressure on the gallbladder
- Nausea or vomiting
- Gallstones
- Constipation
- Tiredness in morning—and feeling better later in the day

## Gallbladder Saved Following Visceral Manipulation

Morag's son had been a patient of mine for a few months. While treating him I had found a restriction around his gallbladder and had released this for him. When he returned for his next visit he told me he had found he could better digest fatty foods and felt less bloated. I explained that this was not surprising, as the gallbladder stores bile, a digestive liquid that does the same job that dishwashing liquid does, in that it breaks down fat in the digestive system. When the gallbladder loses some of its function it is less able to do this, and hence the struggle to eat fatty foods. During the conversation Morag's son mentioned that his mother also had gallbladder problems. She was waiting to have her gallbladder removed, after suffering right-sided pain and having a scan that had shown lots of small gallstones.

He referred his mother, Morag, in to see me. Her surgery was scheduled in eight weeks' time. (One of the benefits of the waiting lists for non-urgent surgery in the UK is that it gives patients time to find other, less-invasive solutions to their health conditions.) When I first saw Morag she showed me a copy of the letter her doctor had written confirming the presence of a large number of small stones in her gallbladder.

When I assessed Morag, I found her gallbladder had restrictions around it and it had lost its Motility. Additionally, the sphincter of Oddi, which is at the end of the tube from the gallbladder into the duodenum, was "frozen"—that means it was not able to do its job of opening and closing appropriately to respond to digestive changes. Morag also had some restrictions in her bowel. Over three sessions I treated her gallbladder and digestive system to restore normal movement and balance. I also gave her advice to drink apple pectin to soften the stones, and to avoid fatty foods. Morag reported that she had passed a number of gallstones with bowel movements and was wondering if she still needed the surgery.

When Morag went for the surgery, eight weeks after I first met her, I suggested she should ask for a rescan just to check it was still necessary. They did rescan her and the report was that there was no evidence of stones. They thought her results from the first scan must have been misread!

Of course, not every case of gallstones can be resolved like this, and in Morag's case she was lucky, as the stones were still small enough to pass. It has now been five years since I treated Morag, and although I have not seen her since, her son reports that she is still doing well. She has had no recurrence of her gallbladder issue. Morag is one of a growing group of about twenty patients I have treated that have managed to avoid gallbladder surgery thanks to VM.

---

## Pancreas

The pancreas actually is composed of two parts. One part is the digestive part, which was discussed above, and produces and releases about 3 to 4.5 pints (1.5 to 2 l) of digestive enzymes into the duodenum per day. The other part is a hormonal part, which is well known for regulating blood sugar by releasing insulin and another hormone, known as glucagon, into the bloodstream. When this mechanism is dysfunctional, diabetes is the result. Given that diabetes is now the fourth leading cause of death in the United States, accounting for about one hundred eighty thousand deaths per year, the importance of the hormonal functions of the pancreas cannot be disregarded.

The pancreas is oblong but has a pointy tail attached that heads off up toward the left side, toward the spleen at a thirty-degree angle. It is a fragile organ, having a texture like thick porridge. It sits in the middle of the duodenum, in the center of the body just above the navel. (See Figure 8.20.) It is connected to the duodenum by the pancreatic duct, which joins the duodenum at the sphincter of Oddi, along with the common bile duct.

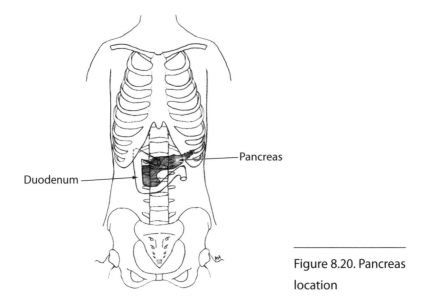

Figure 8.20. Pancreas location

Digestive enzymes enter the digestive system at the pancreatic duct. The pancreas lies in front of the left kidney and the adrenal gland, the common bile duct, the aorta, the inferior vena cava, and several other important blood vessels. It lies behind the stomach and, obviously, has relationship with the duodenum. (See Figure 8.21.) Tissue bridges also attach it to the large intestine and spleen. It is hard not to notice how interconnected all of the structures are in the body.

As the pancreas is a fragile organ, no Mobility treatment is done directly on it. If the pancreas is restricted against a neighboring organ, it is more likely that a practitioner will treat the other organ to benefit the pancreas. However, Motility of the pancreas is checked and assisted, which will usually be done with the practitioner placing one hand over the pancreas with the fingers pointing up toward the left lower ribs. (See Figure 8.22.) The sphincter of Oddi may need to be treated to allow the pancreatic duct to function normally. Treatment will not resolve diabetes, but it may improve the overall well-being of the diabetic person.

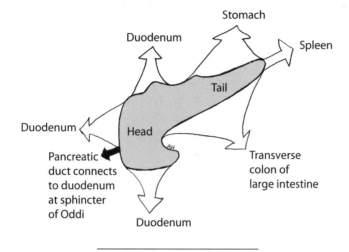

Figure 8.21. Pancreas relations

Possible causes of pancreas issues:

- Duodenum restrictions
- Stomach issues
- Left kidney restrictions
- Spleen issues
- Unbearable grief
- Alcohol consumption
- A diet high in refined sugar

Symptoms of pancreas issues that may improve with VM:

- Back pain in the mid-back area, primarily on the left
- Left-sided low back pain
- Left-sided shoulder pain
- Unexplained thirst
- Feeling hungry just after a meal or craving sweet or fatty foods

- Feeling exhausted after drinking alcohol

- Digestive issues, especially after sweet or fatty foods

- Feeling unwell, especially one to three hours after eating; often involves sweating, fatigue, and nausea

- Cannot stand strong smells, such as perfume

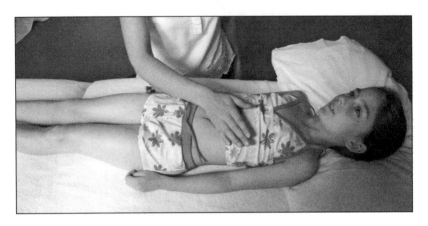

Figure 8.22. Pancreas Motility

### Sphincters

As previously described, the sphincters are valve-like structures that control the rate substances pass from one location to another. There are five of them that concern us in the digestive tract. (See Figure 8.23.)

1. The first one is found at the top of the stomach *(cardiac sphincter)* and controls the reflux of the stomach contents into the esophagus. If this sphincter is not functioning properly, heartburn, or reflux, often occurs.

2. Then there is one at the exit of the stomach, known as the *pyloric sphincter,* which controls the rate and timing of the food passing out of the stomach. It takes around forty minutes for the food to reach this point after someone eats. As discussed above, the stomach is a

little bit like the main wash cycle in the washing machine. For this reason the food needs to be kept in the stomach until this cycle is complete and the stomach has broken down the food as much as is possible at this stage.

3. There is another sphincter at the point where the common bile duct and pancreatic ducts pass into the duodenum, known as the *sphincter of Oddi.* This sphincter controls the flow of the digestive fluids from these ducts into the duodenum.

4. There is a sphincter between the duodenum and the rest of the small intestine, known as the *duodenal-jejunal junction.*

5. The fifth valve of concern here is at the end of the small intestine leading into the large intestine and is known as the *ileocecal valve,* which the food reaches about five to six hours after having been eaten.

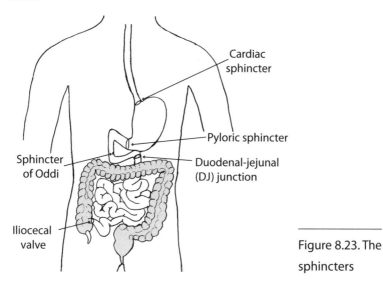

Figure 8.23. The sphincters

Together these sphincters manage the rate of passage of the digested food from one stage to the next, rather like the timer on a washing machine, ensuring that each phase is complete before the food moves on. If these sphincters get out of balance, it can lead to digestive dysfunction.

The sphincters are commonly addressed in VM. Indeed Jean-Pierre Barral has stated that if he could only treat one thing, it would be the sphincters because they have a calming effect on the entire digestive system. The sphincters, like organs, each have a Motility, and their Motility is in a circular fashion. This Motility allows a practitioner to check if the sphincters are functioning normally, and if not, to encourage them to do so. Practitioners may use a direct, indirect, or Recoil technique locally on the dysfunctional sphincter to bring it back into normal function. It is not uncommon for the sphincters to make gurgling noises as they release. Additionally, the patient often will feel a reduction in tenderness and find digestion easier after sphincter treatment. The sphincters have a tendency to function as a team, so usually a practitioner will check and balance all five sphincters listed above.

Possible causes of sphincter issues:

- Bowel diseases—flare-ups of Crohn's, ulcerative colitis, and irritable bowel disease
- Digestive issues, including constipation or diarrhea
- Pregnancy
- Changes in hormonal levels
- Surgery
- Anxiety and stress
- An imbalance of one of the other sphincters

Symptoms of sphincter issues that may improve with VM:

- Digestive dysfunction—gas, belching, poor digestion, reflux
- Bowel diseases: flare-ups of Crohn's and irritable bowel diseases
- Digestive problems during pregnancy

- Digestive issues with menopause
- Digestive dysfunction after surgery
- Feeling anxious, talking a lot
- Stress—treatment helps circulation and nerve supply in abdomen and calms stress response

### *Constipation, Heartburn, and Low Back Pain with Pregnancy*

Elspeth was six months pregnant with her first child when she came in to see me complaining of low back pain, heartburn, and constipation. Constipation is a common challenge during pregnancy, as the mother's body is affected by the growing baby pressing on her bowel or on the nerves and blood vessels that supply it. In pregnancy, heartburn often results when the baby pushes up under the mother's stomach; hence, the valve at the top of the stomach (cardiac sphincter) has the tendency to become dysfunctional. Low back pain is also a regular feature in pregnancy, as the woman's body carries the extra weight of the baby and the additional fluids.

With pregnancy, the soft tissues of the mother's body all become looser. This is due to the hormonal changes she experiences, and the looseness is to allow her body to stretch both with her growing baby and during delivery. This means that Mobility techniques are usually avoided, and in preference, Motility techniques are used.

Using General Listening I was taken to Elspeth's lower right abdominal area. Using Local Listening I found this to be her ileocaecal valve. When I Listened to the valve itself, I found it was dysfunctional. This means it was not correctly carrying out its function of opening and closing in response to the digestive requirements, which could lead to her constipation. I then went on to assess her other sphincters, and found her sphincter of Oddi and cardiac sphincters were also dysfunctional. With Inhibition I confirmed that the ileocaecal valve was the primary restriction.

Using a direction of ease technique I followed the ileocaecal valve into a rotation Motility and then added a small Induction. This allowed the valve to release, and it let out a gurgling noise. I then rechecked the other sphincters and found the other two had corrected. This group release is common, as the sphincters function as a team, and when the primary dysfunction is corrected, the others often also correct.

I saw Elspeth again two weeks later. She reported she had significantly less constipation and heartburn, and that her low back pain had improved, despite her increasing size.

9

# Waterworks

Water is vital for human survival. Without water and a function-ing waterworks system people can only survive for about two weeks—but even less time if the temperature is high or they are exercis-ing. By the time someone is seventy, he or she will have easily drunk over 11,000 gallons (50,000 l) of water, which will all have been processed by the kidneys and bladder. Therefore it is essential that this system is functioning effectively.

The main organs involved in processing water in the body are the kidneys and bladder. They are connected by the ureters, which are pipes that run from each kidney into the bladder. Then from the bladder there is another, shorter pipe, called the urethra, which allows urine to leave the body. (See Figure 9.1.) The main function of the system is to help maintain the composition, volume, and pressure of the blood by removing and restoring water.

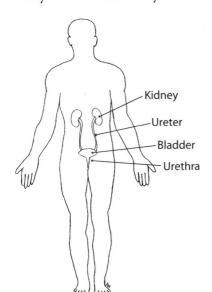

Kidney

Ureter

Bladder

Urethra

Figure 9.1. Overview of the waterworks system

## Kidneys

The kidneys have the function of maintaining the correct fluid balances in the body, by filtering the blood. The kidneys filter more than 450 gallons (more that 1,500 l) of blood each day, with each kidney containing one million individual filters. The kidneys are responsible for filtering the waste products and excess fluid out of the blood; from this a person gets 2 to 4 pints (1 to 2 l) of urine daily. The kidneys clean out the entire blood system every twenty-four hours. The importance of this is that they maintain a person's blood pressure, blood volume, blood concentration, and its pH (acid or alkaline) balance. The kidneys also have some hormonal functions in relation to production of red blood cells, pain, digestion and absorption, and use of calcium. While the kidneys only weigh about a one hundred forty-fourth of the entire body weight, they use about twenty percent of the oxygen, which shows how hard they do work.

The kidneys are located under the diaphragm toward the back and top of the abdomen, behind the peritoneum, which is the lining of the abdomen. (See Figure 9.2.) This means the kidneys move a lot with breathing (up to 1.25 inches, or about 3 cm each breath). Given that a person breathes twenty thousand times per day, each kidney should move about 550 yards (600 m) per day. The right kidney sits a little lower than the left, as the liver takes up so much space on the right. The kidneys are about 4 to 5 inches (10 to 12 cm) long, 2 to 3 inches (5 to 7 cm) wide, and 1 inch (2.5 cm) thick. They are shaped like kidney beans. People have two kidneys, and although anatomically they seem the same, they do have different relations due to the structures surrounding them, and their nerve and blood supplies. The right kidney is known as the digestive kidney, being more involved in the process of digestion, while the left one is known as the genital kidney, being more associated with reproductive or genital issues.

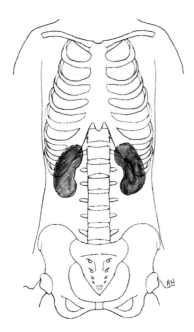

Figure 9.2. Kidney location

The kidneys are not easy to feel. Usually a practitioner will start about the level of the navel from the front and feel through all the tissue layers deep into the abdomen and up toward the ribs to find the bottom part of the kidney. He or she may do this with the patient in a back-lying or a sitting position. The practitioner may also use one hand to press from the back toward the front to bring the kidney forwards a little. He or she will be interested in how the kidneys are able to move in relation to the organs around them. They should be able to slip like wet bars of soap against their neighboring tissues. The practitioner will evaluate whether a kidney has dropped at all, a condition known as ptosis. This is common with kidneys, as they do not have a strong ligamentous support system. Their suspension in the body is assisted by the negative pressure of the chest cavity compared to the abdominal cavity and its sufficient abdominal muscle tone. The kidneys are contained and protected within fatty wrapping. Additionally, because they are fairly solid, they are often affected by trauma shock waves. If they have dropped at all this can impact their functioning, as dropping often results in a strain on the blood vessels that supply the kidneys. This leads to a drop in the amount of oxygen reaching them, which means they cannot work as hard.

The goal of treatment will be to allow the kidney to move more easily in relation to the structures surrounding it. This is vital, considering the effect movement (especially of the diaphragm) has on kidneys. It they are unable to move down with each in-breath, then every breath just compresses the organ; that is a lot of additional force for a restricted kidney. It has been found that in the case of a kidney that has ptosis (dropped), it is more important to improve movement than to be concerned about its position. Often a kidney will gradually return to its normal position in the weeks or months following treatment. In some cases it may never reach its original position but its functioning will recover. Commonly, when treating the kidneys a practitioner will use the breath and leg movements to aid release. This is because they lie so close to the diaphragm and are so greatly affected by breath. Also they sit just in front of the psoas muscle, which is activated by leg movements. After the kidney has been released, the practitioner will usually balance the kidneys' Motility with one another. (See Figure 9.3.)

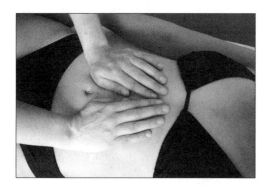

Figure 9.3. Kidney Motility

Possible causes of kidney issues:

- Falling on the coccyx (tailbone) or ribs
- Severe physical trauma (such as a car accident)

- Losing weight too quickly, which affects the fatty pockets
- Childbirth
- Surgery
- Chronic coughing
- Urinary infections and kidney stones
- Colitis or intestinal spasms
- Sedentary lifestyle—too long sitting or standing
- Excessive traveling—e.g., in planes or cars
- Deep fear
- Shock
- Feeling weak or depressed

Symptoms of kidney issues that may improve with VM:

- Intense early-morning or late-night thirst, sometimes enough to wake a person up
- Hunger on arising, sometimes giving way to tiredness and nausea
- Low back pain on wakening, improving soon after getting up, but deteriorating later in the day and disappearing soon after going to bed
- Thigh or knee discomfort, increasing during the day
- Headache due to dehydration
- Sciatica, in some cases
- Left-sided neck pain or restriction
- Mid-back pain or restriction
- Muscular weakness
- Darkened or cloudy urine
- Swelling due to fluid retention
- Intense itching, especially of the legs

- Deep fatigue
- Symptoms worse at end of day
- Cannot tolerate wearing narrow belts
- Indigestion, with a slow transit of food through the digestive system
- Blood pressure issues or variations
- Low back pain relieved by lying down
- Flaky, dry skin

## *Leg Pain with Exercise*

Alisdair was a man who came to me with long-term low back pain and left hip and thigh pain upon exercise. With General Listening I found that I was taken to an area just below his ribs on the left side. With Manual Thermal Evaluation and Local Listening I was able to determine that it was his left kidney that was the primary concern. Once I had explained this to Alisdair I began treatment with him.

His left kidney had ptosis (loss of its normal position), and from my anatomical knowledge, I was aware this could lead to symptoms in the low back and leg due to the fact the kidney sits in front of the psoas muscle. The psoas muscle shortens to support the kidney and prevent it from falling lower. The kidney needs to be able to move over the muscle, and if it cannot, a common result is leg or low back discomfort. The focus of my treatment was to allow the kidney to regain its normal movement and help it move in relation to the muscle.

So I could treat him, Alisdair was lying on his back with his knees bent. I located his left kidney and cupped the lower part of it in the palm of my hand. I then asked him to breathe slowly, following the kidney up toward the diaphragm on exhalation and supporting it there during inhalation. I then asked Alisdair to push his bent left knee toward his chest into my hand to contract the psoas muscle. Doing this allows the kidney to slide over the psoas muscle and create release of its restrictions. I went on to balance the Motility of the kidneys.

Alisdair greatly improved after this session and his low back pain of many years' duration reduced. I treated him three more times before his last symptoms abated. This was a case where a restriction with an organ led to pain that feels like it was due to structural issues, but really had an internal organ cause.

---

## Bladder

The bladder is a hollow organ situated in the pelvis, in front of the vagina in women and the rectum in men. It looks like an upside down fig. Jean-Pierre Barral is very keen that it should not just be dismissed as a reservoir, but rather nicknames it the "little kidney," as he feels it is an equal partner with the kidneys in the waterworks system. They all communicate and are interdependent. The bladder wall is formed of lots of folds so that it can expand to hold urine and collapse when it empties. It is filled with the urine that flows down the ureters from the kidneys. Once full enough, the sphincter, which is like a valve at the bottom of the bladder formed from muscle layers, relaxes, and a person passes urine via the urethra. The bladder can hold 1 to 1.25 pints (400 to 600 ml) of urine, but a person gets the urge to urinate at 0.5 pint (200 ml). When full, the bladder is roughly the size of a grapefruit. Its function is to collect and then excrete urine, and thanks to it, people do not need to spend the whole day on the toilet.

The bladder lies right behind the pubic bone. (See Figure 9.4.) Below it are the pelvic floor muscles and above it is a ligament called the urachus, which runs up to the navel. The muscles underneath the bladder form a valve round the base of the bladder, which allow us to control our urge to urinate. When these muscles relax a person will urinate, there should be no need to push urine out. Therefore when VM practitioners treat the bladder they may work up from the pelvic floor or from the navel down to behind the pubic bone. (See Figure 9.5.) They may also stretch the ureters, the tubes that connect the kidneys to the bladder, as these can be a point of blockage or strain. (See Figure 9.6.) With Motility, often practitioners not only treat the bladder but also balance Motility of the bladder with the kidneys.

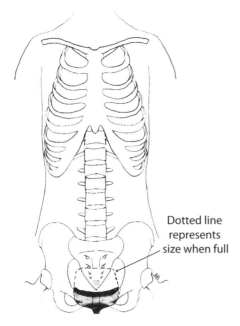

Dotted line represents size when full

Figure 9.4. Bladder location

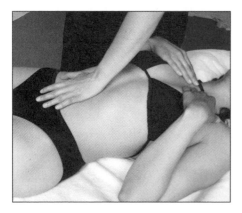

Figure 9.5. Bladder treatment

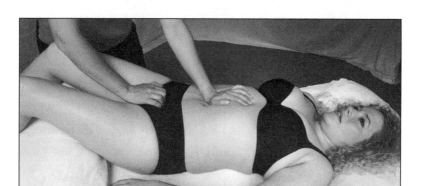

Figure 9.6. Ureter stretch

Possible causes of bladder issues:

- Pregnancy or childbirth
- Constipation
- Falling on tailbone, or low back trauma
- Surgeries
- Pressure from other abdominal organs
- Pelvic infections
- Obesity
- Retroverted uterus (uterus tipped back so it drags bladder down)
- Feeling of need to hold on to keep control

Symptoms of bladder issues that may improve with VM:

- Stress or urge incontinence
- Recurrent or frequent urinary tract infections
- Bed-wetting in children
- Cystitis including interstitial cystitis
- Pain during intercourse in women often following childbirth
- Bladder prolapse

## *Bed Wetting Problem Resolved with Visceral Manipulation*

Caitlin was a six-year-old girl who wet the bed. She had been dry from the age of two to three and a half, and then seemed to lose bladder control again.

I evaluated Caitlin's body with General Listening, Local Listening, and Manual Thermal Evaluation to find that I was pulled into her sacrum, or tailbone, and low back area. So I started treating this area. I asked her mother if she had fallen or injured her low back area. Her mother remembered that she had fallen out of a loft and landed on her back about the age of three and a half.

I treated her low back, then balanced her bladder and its supporting structures in the pelvic area, and then her kidneys. The nerves that supply the bladder seemed to have been affected by her accident. Some of the nerves to this area come from the sacrum, and this was the structure that was restricted when I first met Caitlin.

Gradually, over a six-month period with regular treatment, Caitlin became dry at night and was able to stop using her disposable pull-up pants. She was even able to go to sleepovers at friends' houses.

Visceral Manipulation techniques can be very effective with children. It is most rewarding to see changes in this population. I often think that with their lifetime ahead of them, resolving issues that perhaps affect their development, social life, or family at this stage can have a huge impact on them for life. The effects of VM on them could outlive me!

# 10

# Breathing

The breathing process can be defined as the passage of air through the mouth and nose via the trachea and bronchi, which are the pipes that carry air into and out of the lungs. When considering breathing, one needs to be aware that the rib cage and diaphragm play a large role in breathing. (See Figure 10.1.) If they are not functioning correctly then breathing optimally is not going to be possible. For that reason, in addition to the actual breathing structures, there will be a discussion of the rib cage and diaphragm here.

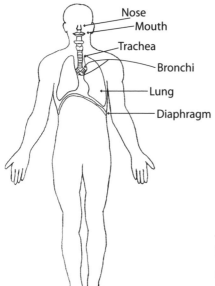

Nose
Mouth
Trachea
Bronchi
Lung
Diaphragm

Figure 10.1. Overview of breathing system

The function of breathing is to allow gaseous exchange to occur by bringing oxygen into the body and helping the removal of carbon dioxide. Humans require oxygen for life—it is required by every cell of every tissue and organ to allow functioning. It is also important for bodies to be able to release the waste product carbon dioxide. If people are locked in a completely sealed room, they will die of carbon dioxide poisoning before they will die of oxygen deprivation.

## The Breathing System

Air is taken into the lungs via the nose and mouth and then down the trachea into the bronchi. The lung structure is composed of many thin membranous bags, known as alveolar sacs. These sacs increase the internal surface area inside the lung and allow a maximum amount of oxygen from the air to be taken into the blood for transport to the cells of the body. The lungs contain 300 billion capillaries (tiny blood vessels)—if they were laid end to end, they would stretch 1,500 miles (2,400 km). About 15 pints (7 l) of air enter the lungs every minute. Of that, 10 pints (5 l) reach the alveoli but only 0.75 pint (350 ml) of oxygen actually go into the bloodstream (five percent of the original volume). However, that excess air is not wasted. Another important function of the lungs is to create a negative pressure, which helps to support the contents of the abdomen and head. This negative pressure creates a type of suction, which helps reduce the true weight of organs, such as the liver. This is the purpose of the excess air that is inhaled.

During breathing, there are two phases, known as inspiration and expiration; each cycle happens about fourteen times per minute. During the day a person breathes in and out about twenty thousand times, meaning any related restrictions will be greatly irritated by the continuous breathing.

Inspiration is an active phase, which means that muscles have to actively contract to allow the air to move into the lungs. The diaphragm contracts and descends to increase the capacity of the chest. The muscles of the chest wall pull the ribs and breastbone (sternum) upward and outward. The soft tissues of the chest, such as the pleura (the sacs around the lungs), and the lungs themselves are very elastic and stretch during inhalation. This causes the air pressure within the alveoli of the lungs to become less than atmospheric pressure, so air is sucked into the lungs.

Expiration is the passive phase, where all the above muscles relax, and the chest size reduces as ribs and breastbone (sternum) move in and down. The lungs reduce in size and the whole process is aided only by the contraction of abdominal muscles and small rib muscles.

The lungs themselves have a spongy or porous texture and would float in water. They are contained in a bag-like structure called the pleura, which is a double-layered membrane. This membrane is very smooth and has fluid between the layers to allow it to gently glide over itself. The lungs' pleura are suspended from the spine in the neck and the first rib. They line the chest cavity and link into the peritoneum, which is the fascia of the abdominal cavity and was discussed earlier in the book. Because of this link, restrictions of the pleura can affect organs in the abdominal area, such as kidneys and liver. The outer layer of pleura lines the inside of the chest wall. The inner layer encapsulates the lungs themselves, covering not only the outside of the lungs but also running between each of the lobes. (See Figure 10.2.) The lungs are divided into lobes (or parts). On the right there are three lobes—the upper, middle and lower lobes, and on the left only two lobes. The function of the lobes of the lungs appears to be to allow better motion during breathing and to help contain any pathology, which would preserve some breathing function even if one part of the lungs was not working properly. The functioning of the lungs and the heart cannot be totally separated, due to their anatomical proximity and also the fact that the heart is the pump that drives the blood flow through the lungs to allow gaseous exchange. For that reason your practitioner may also consider the circulation along with breathing issues.

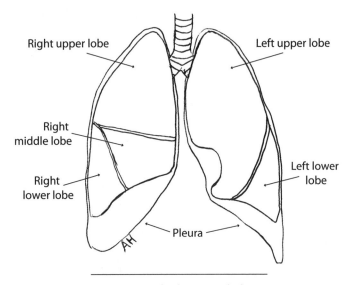

Figure 10.2. The lungs and pleura

The lungs are contained within the rib cage. (See Figure 10.3.) The only place that a practitioner can feel them directly is through the pleura behind the first rib. The lungs extend down to the diaphragm, which

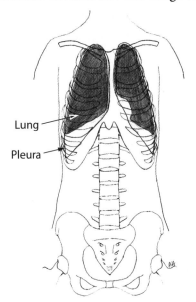

Figure 10.3. Lung location

varies in height with breathing but is usually roughly at the level of the sixth through the tenth ribs.

As with all issues, a practitioner will be Listening to a patient's body and treating what he or she finds. The Listening in relation to a breathing issue may take place far removed from the chest area. However, if taken to the chest area, the VM practitioner will work mostly through the ribs. This means the practitioner will consider the movement possibilities of the ribs, breastbone (sternum), collarbones (clavicles), neck, spine, and the muscles and fascia that cover these areas. The practitioner may also address any restrictions of the trachea, or windpipe, and treat the throat area, as any tensions here could pull into the lung area and restrict breathing. Additionally, he or she may need to consider the heart and circulation and release restrictions within these to allow normal breathing to return. With increased rib cage elasticity a practitioner is able to use pressure to work through the ribs and reach the pleura. Mostly treatment involves addressing the pleura (which is a type of fascia) using Motility Induction directly with the lung tissue.

Practitioners may help to renew slide and glide between two lobes of the lungs in the pleura, or perhaps between the pleura and the sac that surrounds the heart, which is called the pericardium. Additionally they may free up the area called the hilum, where the vessels of the lungs such as arteries and veins enter the pleura, to allow better circulation and hence improve lung functioning. However, as with all organs, not all chest issues result in breathing changes or localized problems. For example, to reach for something in a high cupboard a person needs good shoulder movement, but also the internal organ anatomy has to be mobile. This includes having freedom and smoothness of movement between chest tissues such as the pleura and the diaphragm. (See Figure 10.4.)

Some important nerves that run into the chest area need to be considered. One of these is the phrenic nerve, which supplies the diaphragm. Through nerve manipulation techniques restrictions can be treated, thereby improving diaphragm function and breathing.

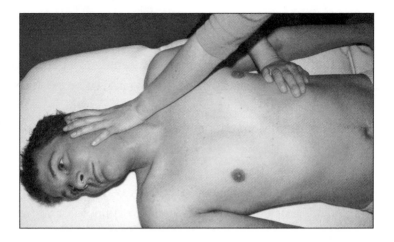

Figure 10.4. Pleural release

Possible causes of breathing issues:

- Trauma either to the chest or neck locally, or general trauma leading to pressure changes
- Surgeries, either on the chest or other areas
- Pollutants from smoking or inhaling chemicals
- Allergies
- Restrictions with other organs
- Issues from development or birth leading to breathing issues or chest trauma
- Infections—chest infections, colds and throat infections, whether of bacterial, fungal, or viral cause
- Tumors
- Problems with abdominal organs, such as the liver or digestive system
- Lack of self-confidence
- Fear of confrontation
- Fear of being dominated or suffocating

Symptoms of breathing problems that may improve with VM:

- Breathing difficulties
- Coughing or sneezing
- Voice changes or crackling
- Noisy breathing
- Pain with breathing
- Backache in the shoulder-blade region or side
- Neck pain and stiffness (because the pleura of the lungs are suspended from the spine in the neck area)
- Arm issues such as carpal tunnel syndrome due to irritation of the nerves that run to the arm
- Tiredness
- Lack of energy
- Excessive sweating
- Increased heartbeat or pulse
- Bluish-gray tinge to the skin
- Poor posture
- Untimely bouts of aggressiveness due to increased carbon dioxide in the blood

## *Chest Pain*

Fiona was a single mother of an eighteen-year-old autistic boy I treated. While bringing him for his appointment she mentioned that she was worried because she had chest pain when she exercised, which had been an ongoing issue for many years. She was particularly aware of it when shovelling coal, and as the family had a coal-fired boiler driving their heating system, this was a daily concern for her. I suggested she make an appointment and we would see what we could find.

General Listening took me into her chest behind her breastbone. With Local Listening I found the restriction behind her breastbone that was affecting her pleura, which is the bag that surrounds the lung. Fiona was concerned that the chest pain might be a heart problem, although her doctor had checked this and found nothing wrong. With Manual Thermal Evaluation I also noted that there was an emotional imbalance associated with her restriction.

I treated Fiona to remove this restriction by engaging the tissues and allowing them to create release, and balancing up the emotional pattern that related to the restriction. By the end of the session she commented that she felt like she could take a proper deep breath for the first time in months. When she tried shovelling coal again the next day she had no pain and has had no recurrence of symptoms since that time. The reason seemed to be that when she shovelled coal her breathing deepened, and this would lead to a stretching of the pleura, which was causing her the pain. Emotionally, she had become so worried that it led to a tightening of her tissues and further exacerbated the situation.

Jean-Pierre Barral often states that the idea of heart problems is one of people's greatest health fears, with only the fear of breast cancer in women outweighing it. Therefore, when one suffers chest pain it is commonly associated with a lot of fear. Often, I see patients who have chest pain or arm pain and are worried about possible heart issues. While these do of course need to be ruled out, there are many other causes of chest pain that are not sinister and can be easily released with VM.

# 11

# Circulation

One of the most important bodily functions is carried out by the circulatory system (also known as the vascular system). Andrew Taylor Still, the founder of osteopathy, believed the "rule of the artery is supreme." (Quoted in Robert Ward's *Foundations for Osteopathic Medicine,* 2nd edition.) Therefore it is not surprising that Jean-Pierre Barral, as an osteopath, has developed VM to include manual techniques for circulation.

Circulation is composed of a series of pipes that carry blood around the body. The circulatory system carries nutrients and oxygen to and from every organ, muscle, and cell of the body. The pipes are divided into three main types—arteries, veins, and capillaries. The arteries carry oxygen-rich blood away from the heart. The veins carry oxygen-depleted blood from all parts of the body to the heart. The capillaries are found in between the arteries and veins, and form a fine mesh like network that lies close to as many of the tissues and cells as possible.

Circulation is driven by the heart, which is a pump. This drives the blood around the body and through the lungs to pick up oxygen. Without circulation, one cannot survive—it would be like trying to drive a car without fuel. Therefore it is a vital area to be considered in healthcare.

## The Heart—the Pump

The heart is the pump that pushes the blood around the body. It creates its own beat through a series of electrical stimuli and is regulated by the big boss, the brain. It is able to regulate for slight changes in rhythm—when someone sneezes, all the bodily functions stop—even the heart. And the effects of emotion on the heart are well known by all—all people remember how it feels to be stressed or anxious, and be aware of their heart racing. The human heart creates enough pressure to squirt blood a distance of up to 30 feet (10 m). In an average human lifetime, a heart will pump 48 million gallons (180 l) of blood. In a healthy adult, the volume of blood is one-eleventh of the body weight, or between 5 to 6 quarts (4.5 to 5.5 l)—this is the same as the amount of oil used in the average V-8 engine.

There are two phases to each heartbeat—a contraction phase, known as systole, and a relaxation phase, called diastole. Combined, the phases take around a second to occur, with the systole lasting for about eighty percent of that time. The contraction phase pushes the blood out of the heart into the vessels, while the shorter relaxation phase allows the heart to refill and get ready for its next contraction. The heart has a series of valves, which open and close with heartbeats to prevent the blood from back-flowing. If the valves are not functioning as they should, a person may end up with a heart murmur. A pulse is felt when the left part of the heart contracts and sends the blood out into the body.

The heart, like the lungs, is so precious it is wrapped up in its own bag, known as the pericardium, which is composed of two layers. (See Figure 11.1.) These layers have a small space between them, which is filled with a slippery fluid to allow them to slide over each other easily with the beating of the heart.

Pericardium
Heart

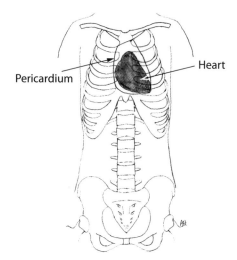

Figure 11.1. Heart location

The outer layer of the pericardium attaches to the breastbone (sternum), the neck, the diaphragm, and the lung pleura. (See Figure 11.2.) The only other support to hold the heart in place comes from the blood vessels. The heart has its own blood supply, which is essential for its functioning. A blockage of one of the coronary arteries could lead to a heart attack.

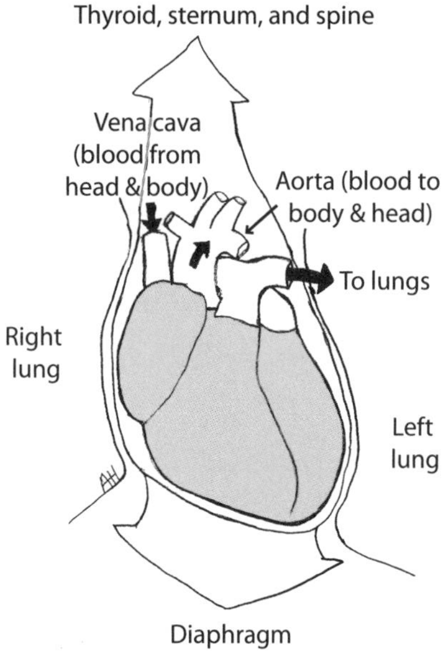

Thyroid, sternum, and spine
Vena cava (blood from head & body)
Aorta (blood to body & head)
To lungs
Right lung
Left lung
Diaphragm

Figure 11.2. Pericardium attachments and relations

The heart is made up of muscle that encloses two separate chambers separated by a fibrous septum. The right side of the heart receives the blood back from the body and sends it on to the lungs to exchange its carbon dioxide for oxygen. The left side pumps the reoxygenated blood that has just been in the lungs to all the cells in the body. It is like a huge one-way system. Each day 1,900 gallons (7,000 l) of blood pass through the heart.

The heart lies on the left side of the body, between ribs two and six. A person's heart is about the size of his or her clenched fist. Its average weight is less than 1 pound (about 300 g in males and about 250 g in females). Because the heart beats about seventy times per minute (that is, one hundred thousand times in a day and more than three billion times in a lifetime), a restriction in the heart or its surrounding tissues can rapidly become aggravated.

Treatment of the heart, like the lungs, involves first addressing restrictions of the rib cage to allow the practitioner to work through the ribs to reach the pericardium, and ultimately the heart itself, its vessels, or its fibrous skeleton. It is possible to manipulate the fibrous structure of the heart. The fibrous structure is the casing of the pump and the valves that control the flow of blood by opening and closing with the heartbeats. (See Figure 11.3.) If this casing is not able to move properly with each heartbeat, then the pump may become less effective. If the coronary vessels (blood vessels that supply the heart) are restricted, then their suppleness can be improved with very specific pressures. Once any restricted tissues are released normal functioning should resume. Often patients feel a great relief from released tension in this area, like a weight has been lifted off their chest.

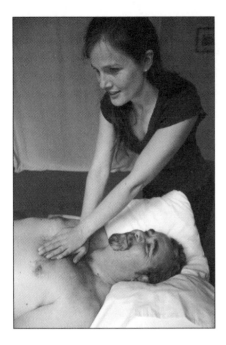

Figure 11.3. Treating the heart's fibrous skeleton

Possible causes of heart issues:

- Trauma to the chest or neck locally, or general trauma leading to pressure changes
- Whiplash; pressure often travels through the heart tissue
- Surgeries, either on the chest or other areas
- Restrictions in relation to other organs
- Issues from development or birth leading to chest trauma
- Developmental problems of the heart (such as the tissues failing to completely close between the sides of the heart)
- Infections
- Smoking
- Dietary issues—too much fat, sugar, or alcohol
- Lack of love or feeling unloved
- Deep distress (e.g., loss of a loved one)

Symptoms of heart issues that may improve with VM:

- Heartbeat or pulse rhythm disturbances, including tachycardia (heart beats too fast), bradycardia (heart beats too slowly), or other heartbeat irregularities
- Imbalances in the pulse from one side to the other
- Shortness of breath for no reason
- Night apnea (tendency to stop breathing when asleep)
- Chest tightness
- Difficulty swallowing or a feeling like the person swallowed something too big
- Pain between the shoulder blades or down the left arm due to viscerosomatic reflexes (organ-to-muscle-pain referral)
- Pain in the jaw or neck, due to viscerosomatic reflexes
- A lasting stitch
- Vertigo or light-headedness
- Extreme pallor
- Sudden anguish or anxiety of no known cause
- The feeling of "Love me; I want some affection"

### Torticollis Due to a Pull on the Pericardium

Kirsty, a woman in her mid-forties, came to me with torticollis, which is a wry (spasming) neck. She had suffered with this for two years following a period of intense stress with her family and work. She had already been to many other professionals for help. Other than having injections of Botox (nerve poison that stops a nerve from functioning for about two to three months) into the muscles of her neck, she had found no relief.

With General Listening I was taken into the area in the center of her chest. With Local Listening I found that it was pulling back through her breastbone into the area at the top of her heart. With my knowledge of tissue types I knew it had a feel of membranes and was about halfway deep into her body. This area was the pericardium. Through my anatomical knowledge I understood that the fascia at the front of the neck actually runs down into the chest and becomes the pericardium (fascia around the heart). A tension in the pericardium can therefore pull on the spinal attachments of fascia, and create neck stiffness and misalignment. For that reason I understood why her body had taken me to her pericardium while her symptoms were in her neck.

Treatment was to release Kirsty's pericardium. I felt how the area from the pericardium up to the neck lengthened under my hands as I worked with her, first using direction of ease and Induction, and then using a little direct stretch to help the fascia find its correct length and tension. I also worked with the fascial layers of the neck to release the upper parts of the line of tension that I could feel.

When I next saw Kirsty she reported that her neck had been substantially better for the first two weeks and then the discomfort had returned a little. All her colleagues, friends, and family had assumed she had just had another Botox injection, as her improvement looked similar what she had following that, which also only lasted a few weeks. I treated her again another three times. With each appointment she had substantial improvement, with some relapse after a few weeks, although each time the relapse reduced in severity. It seemed that her tissues had become so used to being contracted they had a tendency to return to the shortened position. I continue to treat Kirsty every six weeks. Now she has only a slight return of tension between her appointments, so slight that it is not noticeable to her family and friends.

## The Blood Vessels—the Body's Pipes

Arteries are muscular pipes, with smooth muscle in their walls that help push blood along. The muscular action in the artery walls helps blood reach the faraway parts of the body—like the tips of the toes. There are about 65,000 to 100,000 miles (100,000 to 160,000 km) of blood vessels in the adult body—if laid end to end their length would reach two-and-a-half to four times around the earth.

I am sure most people have all found their pulse before, and what they were feeling was an artery. As it is possible to feel arteries, it is through the arteries and heart that VM practitioners can make changes to the circulatory system. Most veins run alongside arteries, so treating the arteries may simultaneously benefit the veins.

Arteries are structured a bit like a tree. (See Figure 11.4.) The largest artery in the body, which is known as the aorta and is about the diameter of a garden hose, leaves the heart and could be considered to be the trunk of the tree. Large branches known as arteries leave the aorta, such as the iliac arteries in the groin and the carotid artery in the neck. Branching off the arteries are smaller vessels known as arterioles, which are like the twigs on a tree.

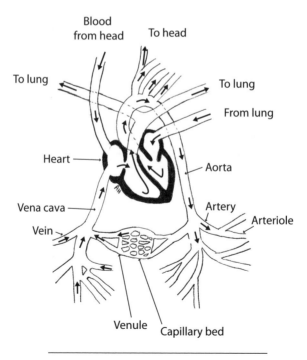

Figure 11.4. Blood circulation in the body

The symptoms of blood vessel problems vary, depending on where the restriction is located. In general, conditions such as cold hands or feet, localized tissue swelling known as edema, a sluggish pulse in one part of the body, and ultimately, conditions such as gangrene are all signs that the circulatory system is not in top form.

## Treatment for the Circulatory System

If Listening takes practitioners to the circulatory system, they will be looking for imbalances and finding ways to help the body release any tension. Where there are matching vessels on each side of your body, they will usually compare pulses from one side of your body to the other. By comparing the pulses, it is possible to see if one side is weaker. If it is, they may start treatment on that side, as artery restrictions will cause a change in the blood flow and hence the feel of the pulse. By feeling your arteries and their pulses it is possible for practitioners to precisely find the part of an artery that is strained and hence help the body to release the restrictions. The balance of vessels from one side to the other is important. Once a restriction has released on one side, practitioners are likely to ensure the other side is fully functional. A tension on one side of the body often creates a strain on the opposite side. The key is that practitioners will use their Listening hand skills to identify where the primary restriction is and precisely encourage your tissues to create release.

Many arteries love to be elongated. Like in a garden hose that has become kinked, the kinks will start to resolve themselves automatically if someone gently supports the end closest to the tap and uses gentle traction to elongate the rest of the hose. It is often the same with blood vessels. Sometimes this is done by adding the movement of a limb to allow the technique to be more effective. (See Figure 11.5.) As with all VM, your practitioner will be facilitating a three-dimensional release and treating in harmony with the intrinsic rhythm of the tissues. Visceral

Manipulation never forces the body or a technique. Once the artery is functioning better, then it may be necessary for a practitioner to address the area supplied by the artery to help restore balance. This can mean treating a patient's organs, or skin rolling.

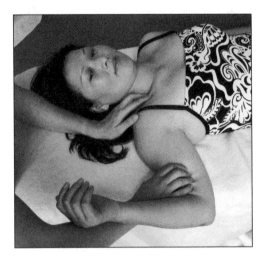

Figure 11.5. Artery treatment

### *Marie-Louise, a Young Lady with Blood Vessel Restrictions*

During a trip to South Africa I was asked to look at a young woman named Marie-Louise, who was a patient of one of the students in a class on learning visceral techniques. Without knowing any of her story, I assessed the twenty-one-year-old one evening; she brought along her doctor to observe.

Using General Listening I was pulled into her right groin area. With further assessment it became clear that I was feeling a restriction of Marie-Louise's femoral artery, one of the blood vessels that runs down into the leg. When I felt the blood vessel itself, it pulled me up through her arterial system to her aorta and then up into the left side of her neck. Her pulse was significantly weaker in the femoral artery of the right groin than in the left, and also in some of the surface blood vessels in her head on the left side compared to the right. Additionally, I found her right leg movements were significantly less than her left—she could only lift her right leg to seventy degrees up from the table she was lying on, but easily managed more than ninety degrees on the left. Her right leg also did not turn in or out with ease.

I shared my findings with the doctor and her practitioner, and let them feel the reduced pulses. She explained she had very low energy and was unable to run due to pain. She'd had pain in her back and under the front of her ribs since breaking her right collarbone two years previously. She also had a coarctation of the aorta, a developmental condition that means a segment of the aorta is narrowed. Perhaps this partly explained the tension pattern in her blood vessels. For no apparent reason, over the past six months she had started having left-sided headaches, which seemed to be aggravated by stress.

I released the femoral artery in her right groin by using a gentle stretch to help it elongate. I then helped her subclavian arteries in her lower neck area to release and then worked with Motility to allow balance to return through the system. While I was working, the skin of Marie-Louise's upper limbs turned red. She then told me she tended to be bitterly cold, despite the African climate. Additionally, during the session she experienced a recurrence of her abdominal and back pain, which then subsided as the release happened.

Through Listening techniques it was clear there was also an emotional component to the tension in her groin, which I then also addressed. It seemed to come from a period four years previously when she had experienced her first major relationship breakup.

After the treatment, Marie-Louise's leg restrictions disappeared. The pulses in the affected arteries were equal side to side, and when Marie-Louise stood up, she noted that she felt like she could stand up straight and was now standing more on her heels.

The question is, how do the broken collarbone and emotional stress lead to blood vessel problems? It seems that due to her developmental condition, Marie Louise's weakest spot was her arterial system. Her body had coped well with the condition, but probably with growing tension in her body due to stress, and possibly a change of pressure in her blood vessels resulting from the break of her collarbone, Marie-Louise's body was no longer able to compensate for her problems. That was when symptoms appeared.

One week later I met Marie-Louise again. She had suffered no headaches and only had back pain when standing. Her abdominal pain had subsided, and her energy had improved. She also had felt quite emotional during the week, but felt like she gained clarity on her relationship issue in a way she had not felt previously.

It is common for patients to find that symptoms seem to develop without any obvious injury or trigger. In many cases like Marie-Louise's, bodies are able to compensate for tensions that exist in them, finding ways to cope and work around these issues. However, at some point one additional minor tension proves to be the "straw that breaks the camel's back," and systems are no longer able to cope with all the minor tensions. In Marie-Louise's case it could be that her collarbone fracture was just one thing too many for her body to work around. This is a common scenario. Often people say they "just get up in the morning" with debilitating pain, or remark that their back seizes up after merely "picking up a sock," which they do every day. One does not have to have symptoms of a tension for a practitioner to be able to find it and to encourage one's tissues to create release. It makes one wonder how much pain and suffering can be prevented through addressing tensions before they become symptomatic.

12

# Reproductive System

B ecause of the obvious differences between males and females in this area, each gender will be considered separately. (See Figure 12.1.)

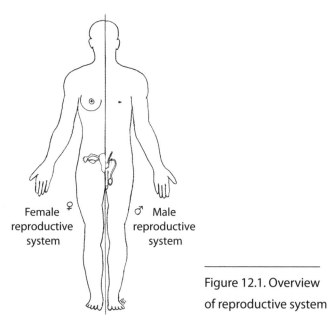

Female ♀
reproductive
system

♂ Male
reproductive
system

Figure 12.1. Overview
of reproductive system

## Female Reproductive System

The internal part of the female reproductive system is composed of the uterus, ovaries, and vagina. (See Figure 12.2.) There are many issues that can develop in regards to the female reproductive system. These include menstruation problems, fertility issues (with as many as thirty percent of American females of child-bearing age now having fertility issues), sexual pain and dysfunction, complaints following childbirth, issues surrounding menopause, prolapses, and hysterectomies. Additionally, the breasts form a part of the female reproductive system.

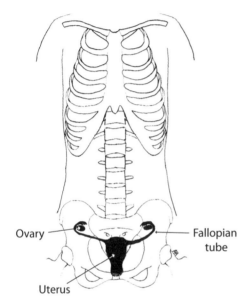

Ovary

Fallopian tube

Uterus

Figure 12.2. Location of female reproductive organs

### Uterus

The uterus is a thick-walled, hollow, muscular organ that is shaped like an upside-down pear. Its function is to hold and protect a growing baby. For this purpose it has to have immense extensibility, and then provide the muscular contractions that will push the baby out when he or she is fully grown. The uterus is also involved with each menstruation, and restrictions of the uterus may lead to pain either at this time or during intercourse.

The uterus is usually 2 to 3 inches (7 to 8 cm) long, about 1.5 inches (4 cm) wide at its widest point, and 1 inch (2 to 3 cm) thick. It weighs from 2 to 4 ounces (60 to 120 g), although this increases to double its size and weight with menses and to one thousand times its normal size, weighing 2.2 to 2.4 pounds (1,000 to 1,200 g) with pregnancy. It is located in the midline of the body, and the top part of it can be felt above the pubic bone. It lies about halfway back through the pelvic area, sandwiched between the bladder in front of it and the rectum behind it. It can be in various positions, bent forward or tipped back. It depends on the pelvic floor muscles and ligaments for stability, with the upper part of the uterus needing to be able to move in situations such as a full bladder or pregnancy.

From the uterus there are also ligaments, which run to each ovary (known as the ovarian and broad ligaments), and the fallopian tubes run from the ovaries to the top of the uterus at each side. Because of these it is impossible to completely separate the uterus and ovaries.

Treatment for the uterus can be done in various ways. A patient may be lying on her back, side, or in an elbow-and-knees position, depending on the exact way her uterus is positioned and on its restrictions. (See Figures 12.3 and 12.4.) The practitioner may also need to treat the patient's pelvis to address any issue of the bony frame that is affecting the pelvic floor tension and hence the tensions around the uterus and vagina. The aims of treatment are to allow release of any restrictions in the tissues around the uterus and help balance tensions of the ligament system that supports it. Generally treatment on the uterus is not carried out during pregnancy or if a woman has an IUD fitted (intrauterine device for contraception), as this may become dislodged. Some practitioners of VM who have done specialist training and are licensed to do so may treat internally to help female reproductive issues. This means they will wear a glove and then work inside the vagina or rectum to reach the lower end of the uterus and the pelvic floor more directly. For some patients this approach may be the only way that the tissues can be reached and treated.

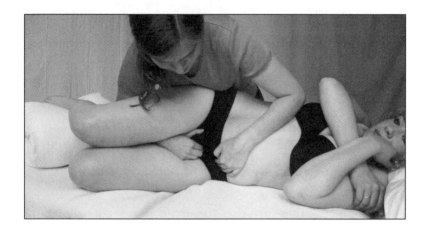

Figure 12.3. Treatment of uterus with patient lying on her side

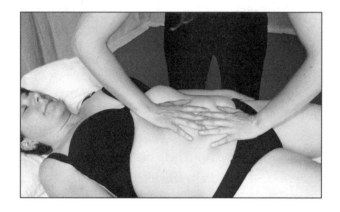

Figure 12.4. Treatment of uterus with patient lying on her back

Possible causes of uterus issues:

- Infections
- Fibroids
- Tumors
- Trauma, such as seatbelt injuries in car accidents or falls
- Hysterectomy

- Childbirth, including Caesarean-section or assisted deliveries
- Pregnancy
- Abnormal uterus position
- Postural changes due to sport or prolonged wearing of high heels
- Any uterus or pelvic surgery
- Ovarian cysts
- Endometriosis
- Emotional issues of various types, including those related to a previous pregnancy, miscarriage, or sexual issues

Symptoms of uterus issues that may improve with VM:

- Lower abdominal pain
- Menstruation problems, including irregular, absent, or painful periods
- Premenstrual Syndrome (PMS)
- Infertility
- Pregnancy issues, including miscarriages
- Varicose veins
- Digestive problems, such as constipation
- Bloating
- Urine problems, such as increased frequency, pain on urination, or incontinence
- Pain in the low back area
- Pain on intercourse or loss of libido
- Uterine prolapse

### *The Ovaries and Fallopian Tubes*

The ovaries are two small grayish-pink oval organs that weigh less than 0.1 ounce (2 to 3 g) each. They are about 1 inch (3 cm) long, 0.66 inch (1.5 cm) wide, and 0.33 inch (1 cm) thick. When a female is born, the ovaries contain around one million eggs, but by the time the woman reaches puberty, there are only about twenty thousand left in each ovary. A woman has forty thousand possible eggs—of which only four hundred will get the opportunity to create a new life, although only a few will ever be fertilized and develop, depending on the size of her family! Eggs are released at the rate of one or two per month; they decompose if they are not fertilized. The ovaries also release reproductive hormones at the time the egg is released. Therefore ovary restrictions can have an impact on the hormonal balances.

The ovaries are attached to the uterus via the ovarian and broad ligaments. There are also ligaments that suspended them from above. The fallopian tube does not actually attach to the ovary but is suspended next to it. The 4.5-inch (12 cm) tube runs from each ovary to the uterus. Its end is funnel shaped. Once an egg is released by the ovary, every one to two months, it moves into this funnel and along the fallopian tube. The ovaries are found just inside the outside edges of the pelvis, about 1 inch (2 cm) above the pubic bone.

Treatment of the ovaries focuses on allowing them to gain more freedom of movement by stretching and releasing the ligaments that attach to them. The ovaries should also have good Motility (their own intrinsic movement) and be in balance with each other. Balance and Motility are typically addressed when the ovaries are treated. (See Figure 12.5.) The fallopian tubes can be elongated to help restore their functioning and reduce any scar tissue that may have built up around them. Mostly these techniques are done when the patient is lying on her back, and like for the uterus, some practitioners of VM may incorporate internal treatment to further release restrictions.

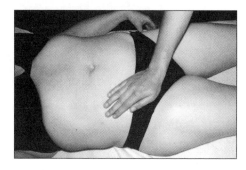

Figure 12.5. Ovary Motility

Possible causes of ovary or fallopian tube issues:

- Surgery, especially of the pelvic or abdomen
- Infections—a tubular infection has the potential to block a tube or create adhesions and affect fertility
- Trauma
- Ectopic pregnancies (that is, pregnancies that happen in the fallopian tube, which often have to be surgically removed)
- Childbirth
- Long-term or severe anxiety leading to tube spasms
- Ovarian cysts
- Endometriosis

Symptoms of ovary or fallopian tube issues that may improve with VM:

- Pelvic pain
- Premenstrual syndrome
- Pain with menstruation, or lack of menstruation
- Low back pain
- Infertility
- Leg or arm pain
- Lower abdominal pain or tension
- Constipation

- Bloatedness of the abdomen
- Weight gain
- Cyclic edema (fluid retention)
- Psychological changes, including hyperanxiety, irritability, or depression

## A New Arrival for a Family

When I first met Iona she was a twenty-eight-year-old mother of a seven-year-old girl. She was happily married and very much wished to have a second child, although she had not been successful in her attempts. She had been through the conventional medical route. She had scans and a laparoscopy that had shown some scarring around her womb and one fallopian tube, but had provided no real explanation. Her only remaining option was to have In Vitro Fertilization (IVF), which she was hoping to avoid.

When I first worked with Iona, General Listening took me to her lower pelvis. With Local Listening and Motility testing I could feel that her womb was pulled to the left side. It was causing a tension along her fallopian tubes. I asked about her delivery of her daughter. It had been very long and had resulted in her daughter having to be pulled out in a hurry. She described the feeling as if they were "pulling out her insides with the baby." Clearly this had resulted in a lot of adhesions.

I treated Iona every three weeks over a six-month period, following the Listening that took me to her womb and fallopian tubes initially, and then followed on to include her ovaries, pelvic floor, and bowel. During this time her menstruation became less painful, and gradually the tensions pulling on her womb reduced. Normal Motility was restored to her womb, and on the last visit I said to Iona I did not think there was much more I needed to do. We agreed to leave it for three months, and then I recheck to see that everything still felt like it was functioning well.

When I saw her three months later I went to the waiting room to meet her and she smiled at me and flipped up her top to show me her stomach. She was seven weeks pregnant. Seven months later she gave birth to another daughter, and I received a large bouquet of flowers.

Not every case of infertility can be resolved with VM, but where mechanical restrictions are causing difficulties, VM may help. This is an example of a structural restriction having an impact on the body's functioning. It is not only infertility that may benefit from VM. I also regularly work with women who have had repeated miscarriages, and am always delighted to have a role in allowing a little person to come into the world.

---

### Breasts

The breasts are a glandular organ whose function is to produce milk. Additionally, breasts play a well-known role in attraction and are regarded as a symbol of femininity. They are held in place by only ligaments and have no muscular component. They are formed of a network of ducts and vessels and connect into the lymphatic glands in the armpits and lower neck. Their nerves are supplied by the same nerves that supply the arm and upper chest area, so confusion is possible between breast, rib, and arm pain.

Breasts are very often the part of the body where women are fearful of having a problem, whereas men are more commonly preoccupied with the heart. Breasts respond to hormonal changes, often becoming more sensitive at ovulation and just before menstruation. Additionally, hormonal treatment such as the oral contraceptive pill or Hormone Replacement Therapy (HRT) may affect breast tissue. While it may be possible to aid nonsinister breast changes with VM, it is suggested that any suspicious signs are carefully examined by a woman's doctor or gynecologist.

Visceral Manipulation assessment of the breasts is often done with Manual Thermal Evaluation. (See Figure 12.6.) The areas of heat projection over the breasts give a clue as to the nature of the breast problem.

Treatment of the area involves assisting the nerves and circulation in the area, along with the fascial connections of the rib cage.

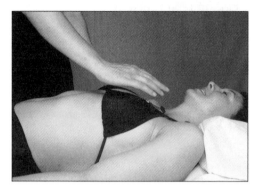

Figure 12.6. Breast evaluation

Possible causes or signs of breast issues:

- Hypersensitivity. This is usual at time of ovulation and running up to menstruation. It is usually a sign of hormonal imbalances, which can be due to liver congestion, a lack of necessary omega-3 oil (found in fish or flax seed), or lack of fiber, all of which aid hormonal breakdown.
- Congestion. The breasts seem larger and heavier. This can be from mechanical causes, such as wearing a bra that is too tight. If it is the same on both sides it is unlikely to be a big problem.
- One breast larger. Very few women have exactly the same size breasts. If this is from the time of formation, it is likely to be due to imbalances of the rib cage and chest area. If this develops suddenly, advice should be sought.
- Lumps. These may be malignant or not. All cysts and lumps require medical investigation to determine their nature.
- Skin changes. If the skin changes on the breast, looking either puckered, drawn in, or like small pits, they must be examined.
- Discharge. Any discharge other than milk with breastfeeding is not normal and needs medical examination.

- Neck, back or shoulder pain. This may be due either to the shared nerve supply between the breasts and these areas or to the weight of the breast tissue and postural changes that can result.
- A women's fear of showing her femininity, or feeling lonely or insecure.

Symptoms of breast issues that may improve with VM:

- Breast congestion
- Breast hypersensitivity
- Neck, back, or shoulder pain
- Feelings of insecurity

## Male Reproductive System

The male reproductive system is composed of the penis, testes, and prostate. (See Figure 12.7.) The purpose of the testes is to create sperm. They manufacture ten million new sperm cells each day—enough to repopulate the entire planet in only six months if they all led to fertilization. The prostate is part of the reproductive system that lies internally in a male. Its function is to secrete a milky fluid that is one component of semen, which then combines with the sperm for ejaculation.

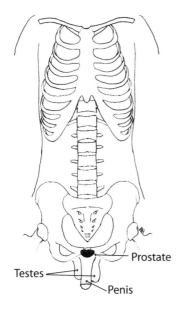

Figure 12.7. Location of male reproductive organs

The prostate is a gland that is about the size of a chestnut, weighing less than 1 ounce (about 20g), located under the bladder. It is reddish-gray in color and fairly solid. The urethra that is the exit from the bladder passes through the prostate, so it is rather like a doughnut ring around the urethra. The prostate is supported by fascia and by the muscles of the pelvic floor. It has several times of growth, one in early puberty when the prostate doubles in size, and then it grows again from ages twenty-five to thirty, and then after the age of forty-five. It is not uncommon for the prostate to become enlarged, especially in older men, and it can end up the size of an orange and reach ten times its original weight. In these cases it may lead to pressure on the bowel or rectum and hence its enlargement may lead to constipation. The prostate is surrounded by a tough capsule, which prevents it from growing too large. Instead it can lead to tightening like a clamp around the urethra. This may result in bladder issues, problems with urination, and erectile dysfunction.

The focus of treatment for the prostate is to ensure that the prostate is able to move normally with the tissues that it lies next to, including the urethra, which passes through it. Once the tissues supporting the prostate are balanced and any restrictions of the pelvic floor released, Motility of the prostate can be addressed. Some VM practitioners may also use internal treatment from the rectum to help soften the gland's consistency and improve the circulation surrounding it. Usually the patient will be lying on his back, possibly with one or both knees bent to allow treatment of his pelvic floor. (See Figure 12.8.) A stretch of the pelvic floor muscles may also be done in a sitting position. It may also be necessary to treat the bony pelvis to balance the tensions around the prostate gland.

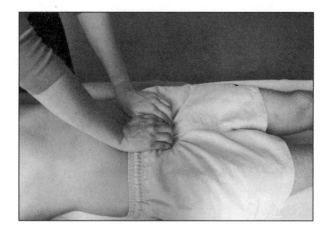

Figure 12.8. Prostate treatment

Possible causes of prostate issues:

- Infection

- Pelvic floor or low back trauma

- Hormone imbalances

- Age-related changes

- Medication (especially over-the-counter cold or allergy medications)

Symptoms of prostate issues that may improve with VM:

- Urinary dysfunctions, including a weak flow, urgency, leaking, or dribbling

- Needing to get up in the night to pass urine

- Inability to urinate

- Erectile dysfunction

- Loss of libido

- Difficulty ejaculating

- Discomfort in the lower abdomen

## *An Accident at Work Leads to Male Sexual Dysfunction*

Cameron complained of pain in his pelvic floor and a need to urinate several times a night. He also reported pain and difficulties maintaining his erection at times, which led to understandable anxiety around intercourse. He had a lack of clarity around his career, feeling that he needed to change careers, as his current one offered few opportunities for promotion, paid poorly, and no longer challenged him. At the same time, he was not feeling motivated to make the changes.

Cameron's General Listening was to his pelvic floor under his prostate. Local Listening confirmed the prostate was involved. While I was treating Cameron he remembered an accident at his last job where he had fallen from a scaffolding rig around 15 feet (4.5 m) high and had come down heavily on the base of his spine. Cameron's prostate felt like it had been pushed up in his body; gradually along with the help of a lot of heat it was able to release and settle back into his pelvic floor.

Over the next few weeks Cameron also started to consider a new career. He arranged to go to night school and started a course in graphic design. Cameron reported that his pain and dysfunction with intercourse greatly improved immediately after treatment and that he also felt his sex drive had improved following the session. He found that many nights he did not have to get up to urinate.

Emotionally, it is important for a man to have a clear position in his life. For Cameron this was not clear, given all his career uncertainty. While I am not suggesting this was the full cause of his prostate concerns, it is possible that this emotional component along with the physical injury contributed to make this prostate issue pressing enough for him to seek treatment.

# 13

# Hormonal System

Hormones form a chemical control mechanism for the body. Many body functions rely on hormones for their coordination and control. Hormones are produced by endocrine glands, which release hormones directly into the body fluids, mainly the blood. Then the hormones travel in the fluids to reach areas of the body that are often a long way from the gland that made them. Therefore hormones can have a more global effect on the body. Most people well know, for example, the effects that premenstrual tension (PMT) can have on women, and in many cases even on their male partners and colleagues!

The endocrine glands are found in various places throughout the body. (See Figure 13.1.) These include the pituitary and pineal glands in the brain, thyroid and parathyroid glands in the neck, pancreas in the middle of the abdomen, adrenals sitting above the kidneys, and testes or ovaries in the pelvis. In addition, there are various other organs that have some hormonal functions, such as the brain, liver, thymus, heart, kidney, stomach, and duodenum. Hormone activity is generally controlled by the nervous system. With VM, the nervous system and circulatory system, which are the usual modes of hormonal transport, are often considered along with the endocrine glands when looking at hormonal issues.

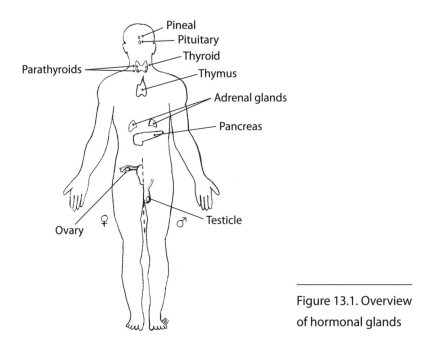

Figure 13.1. Overview of hormonal glands

The hormonal system is like a large orchestra, with the conductor or master level of control being the hypothalamus of the brain. The hypothalamus sends out instructions via the pituitary gland to affect the other organs. In some cases a hormone will be sent out by the pituitary gland into the blood, and it will act as a messenger to tell an organ or tissue to do something. For example, the pituitary gland sends hormonal messages to govern the production of milk in the breast tissue, or to the liver for growth and development. In other cases there is a middleman, so the pituitary hormones start by sending off a hormonal message to another endocrine gland. This then alters the rate of a particular hormone being produced by these glands, such as the thyroid, adrenals, ovaries, and testes (see Figure 13.2). These glands then have an effect on other organs; for example, the thyroid then influences the function of the heart, brain, and cells responsible for growth, development, and tissue repair. The body is amazingly intricate, and so very precise.

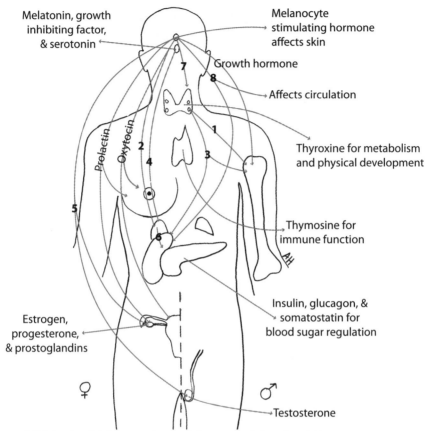

Melatonin, growth inhibiting factor, & serotonin

Melanocyte stimulating hormone affects skin

Growth hormone

Affects circulation

Thyroxine for metabolism and physical development

Thymosine for immune function

Insulin, glucagon, & somatostatin for blood sugar regulation

Estrogen, progesterone, & prostoglandins

Testosterone

Prolactin

Oxytocin

**1** Calcitonin  **2** Adrenocorticotropic hormone  **3** Parathyroid hormone
**4** Angiotensinogen  **5** Follicle stimulating hormone & lutenizing hormone
**6** Aldosterone  **7** Thyroid stimulating hormone  **8** Antidiuretic hormone

*Arrows represent a hormone pathway.*
*Hormones that have a more global effect on the body are noted outside of the body.*

Figure 13.2. Hormone functions in the body

Hormonal messages return to the brain to let the brain know what is happening in the body and whether any hormonal adjustments need to be made. This is known as a feedback loop. It is like the conductor of the orchestra hearing the result of his or her instructions and modifying them if necessary.

Many of the organs listed above also relate to other body systems. Those organs with only partial hormonal function are discussed elsewhere in this book. For example, the pancreas is found in Chapter Eight, "Digestive System," and the reproductive glands (testes and ovaries) are addressed in Chapter Twelve, "Reproductive System." This means that the pineal, pituitary (both located within the brain), thyroid and parathyroid glands, and the adrenals are the only hormonal organs that will be discussed below.

## Hormonal Glands Found in the Brain

The glands that are responsible for hormonal release located in the brain area are the pineal and the pituitary glands.

### Pineal Gland

This gland is shaped like a tiny pinecone and located approximately in the middle of the skull, within the brain tissue. Its function is related to sleep/wake cycles through its release of a hormone, called melatonin. It releases melatonin when it is darker. An imbalance of the pineal gland contributes to insomnia, jet lag, and Seasonal Affective Disorder (SAD). The latter is well known in some places where daylight in the winter months is severely rationed, such as Scotland and Scandinavia. Its main symptom is depression and it is thought to be due to the overproduction of melatonin.

Possible causes or symptoms of pineal issues:
- Insomnia
- Jet lag
- Seasonal Affective Disorder
- Depression or tiredness related to lack of daylight

*Pituitary Gland*

The pituitary gland is a small pea-sized structure of about 0.5 inch (1.33 cm) in diameter. It is attached to a part of the brain known as the hypothalamus via a small stalk. (See Figure 13.3.) The pituitary sits in a small dip in the sphenoid bone (one of the skull bones located behind the eyes), so any restriction of this bone can lead to pituitary tensions.

The pituitary gland is known as the master control gland of the hormonal system, although really it is under the control of the hypothalamus of the brain via nerve connections. When stimulated, the pituitary triggers other hormonal glands to function, including the thyroid, adrenals, ovaries, and testes. Additionally, it leads to the release of hormones that can affect the production of milk in the breast tissue, or in the liver for growth and development.

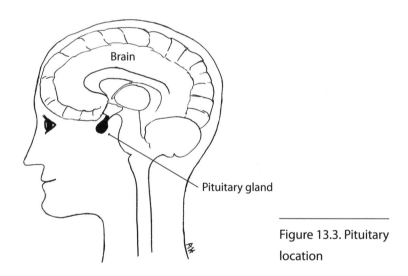

Brain

Pituitary gland

Figure 13.3. Pituitary location

Possible causes or symptoms of pituitary issues:

- Dwarfism (underproduction of growth hormone during development)
- Gigantism (overproduction of growth hormone during development)

- Acromegaly (very large hands, feet, jaw, and soft tissues)
- Change in skin color
- Change in thyroid or adrenal function
- Reproductive hormone imbalances, when extreme leading to possible impotence in males or absence of menstrual cycles in females
- Imbalances in milk production after childbirth
- Breast tenderness
- Blood sugar imbalances

### *Thyroid and Parathyroid Glands*

The thyroid gland is situated in the front of the neck, a bit closer to the top of the rib cage than to the chin. It is shaped like a butterfly that has just flown into the neck, with the two "wings" out toward the sides of the neck and the narrowest part of the gland in the midline. (See Figure 13.4.) It is larger on women than men, and increases in size with pregnancy. Toward each corner of the thyroid gland and embedded into it are the four parathyroid glands. Due to their close anatomical relationship to the thyroid, they will be discussed here.

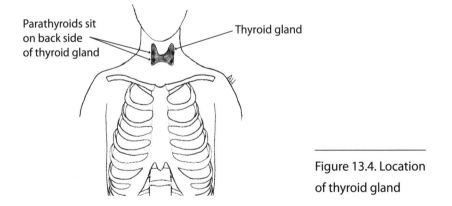

Parathyroids sit on back side of thyroid gland

Thyroid gland

Figure 13.4. Location of thyroid gland

If the thyroid gland gets out of balance it can often lead to very notice-able changes in growth and development. The thyroid governs the rate of metabolism, which is how much energy we have and how much food we require. If the thyroid gland becomes less active it is known as hypothy-roidism. This is when there are not enough of the hormones produced. This results in the metabolic rate slowing down, and from that, ensuing weight gain without any increase in food intake. In addition there may be reduced appetite, mental sluggishness, muscular cramping, chilliness, a slowed heart rate, constipation, and tiredness.

Hyperthyroidism has the opposite effects, causing symptoms such as weight loss, increased appetite, agitation, an increased heart rate, irrita-bility, confusion, sweatiness, feeling too hot, diarrhea, and protruding eyes. The causes of thyroid imbalance are generally caused by the control mechanisms of the thyroid gland, which are through hormones from the pituitary, a deficiency of iodine in the body, or a structural change such as a growth, a nodule or a tumor on the thyroid gland.

The parathyroid glands and thyroid work together to regulate calcium balance in the body. If calcium gets out of balance it can lead to spasms, uncontrollable movements of the muscles, or bone weakness.

As with most other organs, the first consideration with VM is whether the thyroid has freedom to move. If restriction is found, the practitioner may gently treat the patient's thyroid gland itself or the layers of fascia around it—that is, the fascial layers of the neck. The thyroid is a soft, sponge-like organ, and as it is situated close to the surface of the neck, treatment of it is very gentle. (See Figure 13.5.) The thyroid should feel even from side to side to the practitioner. Motility balance techniques may be the treatment of choice.

Treatment of the thyroid can also be via the arteries. The thyroid is supplied by two pairs of arteries—the superior and inferior thyroidian arteries. Jean-Pierre Barral has found that rolling the skin that lies over the thyroid stimulates the nerves that also supply the thyroid gland and can have an effect on thyroid size. As with any organ, tension can lead to

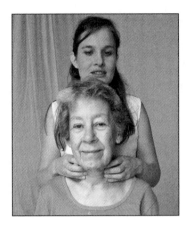

Figure 13.5. Thyroid treatment

changes in the skeletal range of motion and function in the areas it over-lies. In this case, thyroid gland tension can cause changes in structural Mobility or pain in the neck. For a person to bend the neck forward, the visceral components of the neck must be free to glide and slide. As Jean-Pierre Barral said in one of his 2009 class lectures, "The body is not masochistic." In relation to the thyroid that means that if there is a ten-sion of the gland, the body will not allow the person to bend his or her neck forward. The body is preventing the troubled thyroid gland from becoming overly compressed. This leads to a fixation in the viscera in the neck and a reduced range of motion of the neck.

Possible causes of thyroid issues:

- Thyroid goiter or tumor
- Exposure to radiation (kills off thyroid cells)
- Genetic factors
- Severe shock or stress
- Infection
- Trauma to the throat area
- A diet low in iodine
- Pituitary or hypothalamus dysfunction (their hormones regulate the thyroid)

Symptoms of thyroid issues that may improve with VM:

- Being overweight
- Unexplained weight gain
- Being underweight
- Weight loss
- Increased neck size (puffiness)
- Tiredness
- Mental sluggishness
- Bulging eyes
- A change in appetite levels
- A change in heart rate
- Poor temperature regulation
- Diarrhea or constipation
- Premenstrual syndrome
- Menopausal depression
- Irritability
- Guilt—especially family guilt or guilt of a mother

### *Hitting the High Notes*

Sheena was a sixty-three-year-old woman who came to see me to help her singing voice. She had been referred to me by a colleague. Initially I was unsure I would be able to do much for her, given that she had already had CranioSacral therapy from my colleague, and I was assuming this would be the treatment method I would need to use.

As usual I started my assessment with General Listening and Manual Thermal Evaluation, which drew me to Sheena's throat area. With Local Listening I identified a tension in the front of the throat, involving both fascia around the hyoid bone (a small horseshoe-shaped bone just under the chin) and the area of her thyroid gland. The pull through the fascia then went up to the floor of her mouth and around to the base of her skull.

I started treating her using VM techniques to release the fascia at the front of the neck. In this area there are a number of layers of fascia, and both her middle and deep layers were restricted. The techniques involved having Sheena swallow, and gradually the tensions, which were greater on the right side, reduced. I went on to balance tension on the hyoid bone and the occiput (the bone at the base of the skull), and to use Motility Induction on her thyroid, which felt sluggish, especially on Inspir.

While Sheena had not reported any thyroid-related problems, her singing voice did clear and she was able to hit higher notes than she had for the past twenty years. This greatly delighted her, as she had retired and wanted to be able to take part in various choral groups. It was also noticeable that her speaking voice did not sound crackly any more. I treated Sheena for a total of six sessions.

### Adrenal Glands

The adrenal glands sit on top of the kidneys. (See Figure 13.6.) They are the "stress response" glands. Through the hormones released by the adrenals (adrenaline, noradrenalin, cortisol, and other steroids) they contribute to energy balance, repair of damaged cells, fluid balance, and stress response. It is thanks to the adrenals that a person responds to a stressful physical or mental situation by being ready for "fight or flight." When the adrenals release these hormones, the heart rate increases, thereby increasing circulation. Energy production increases, the pupils dilate, the digestive system relaxes, and breathing becomes deeper.

As the adrenals lie deep in the body, it is not possible to treat them directly. Therefore with VM the approach is to ensure freedom of movement of the tissues that surround them, specifically ensuring the diaphragm and kidneys have good Mobility.

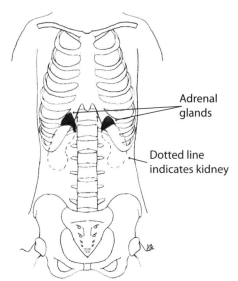

Figure 13.6. Adrenal location

Possible causes of adrenal issues:

- Prolonged or severe stress
- Trauma
- Infection
- Tumor (especially of the adrenals)
- Genetic conditions (such as congenital adrenal hyperplasia)

Symptoms of adrenal issues that may improve with VM:

- Inability to handle stress
- Weight loss and lack of appetite
- Nausea and vomiting
- Increased or reduced blood pressure
- Change in skin coloring
- Change in body fat distribution
- Bruising easily or slow to heal wounds
- Muscular weakness

- Increased infections
- Mood swings

## *A Blow to the Back from Rugby*
## *Results in a Stressed-Out Sheep Farmer*

Blair came to see me complaining of back pain following a rugby game two months previously where he had ended up on the bottom of a scrum. It had collapsed in on him, with another player landing on his back.

General Listening took me to his spine, at the level of his lower rib cage. With Blair lying on his stomach, I then went on to do Local Listening over his spine. This took me to the vertebrae of T9 and T10 (at the lower rib cage, a bit higher than the low back).

I started treatment at this area, releasing the restriction of the spine with a direction of ease and Induction technique. Listening then took me forward in Blair's body to the kidneys and abdominal muscles. I balanced the spine with this area.

The next time I saw Blair he reported that his back pain was much improved, and he had stopped suffering from muscle spasms in his mid-back area. He also commented that he and his wife had both noticed that he had been better able to deal with things in a calm manner since his treatment. He had found over the previous two months that everything seemed to be getting on top of him, even though the stresses on his sheep farm had not altered. I explained to him that the nerve supply from T9 and T10 supplies the kidneys, adrenal glands, and muscles, both in the back and front of the lower rib cage and upper abdominal area. Therefore his injury could have affected the nerve supply to his adrenals and hence his stress-handling abilities.

# 14

# Immune System

The immune system can be compared to an internal army that is waiting to fight any invaders. The system responsible for the body's defense is the lymphatic system. This is a fluid system composed of vessels, nodes, and some organs. The lymphatic system is linked into the circulatory system; therefore the circulation will often be treated along with any immune system problems. There are various main camps for the army within the lymphatic system, these being the spleen, thymus, appendix, patches in the small intestine known as Peyers patches, and the tonsils. The lymphatic system is a series of pipes but without a pump of its own. It relies on the movement of its muscular walls, of surrounding structures, and of the circulatory system to move fluid within it. The lymph nodes contain valves, which make sure the lymph fluid is moving only in the correct direction. They also filter foreign invaders out of the fluid, trap them, and then allow them to be destroyed—this is the reason people may experience swollen lymph nodes when they are ill.

Tonsils and appendixes are perhaps most famous for being removed. Neither of these is essential for survival, although the effects of their removal and the compensations the body goes through after their removal are unclear. However, what is known is that both, along with Peyers patches located on the small intestine, function as part of our immune system. It seems that tonsils are located to "catch" infections we swallow or breathe in. The appendix, a finger-like projection from the cecum (part of the large intestine) of about 3 inches (8 cm) long, seems to have immune functions in relation to digestion. Recently, there is evidence to suggest that the appendix releases a chemical that helps digest raw meat and kill off any infections it carries, something that our distant ancestors may have required more than modern people do. Peyers patches are there to prevent bacteria entering the bloodstream from the small intestine. There is no further discussion of these tissues in this book, except to say they would be influenced along with treatment of the digestive system structures of which they are part. The spleen is discussed in more detail below.

Given that people are continuously surrounded by infection, the immune system does a remarkable job at preventing illness. People rely on the immune system to fight infections, meaning that they generally get rid of an infection within a few days of being affected by it. Considering that places where the hands often rest, a desk or table, for instance, are likely to have approximately ten million bacteria, the immune system must be considered an exceedingly strong and effective army.

## How the Immune System Works

People come into contact with millions of infections every second, be it via things the skin touches, the ones the lungs breathe in, those that enter via the mouth with food and drink, or those that reach the urinary or genital systems. There is a continuous system patrolling around the body, composed of various immune cells. These cells check out the invaders and destroy them when possible. However, when either the invader is unrecognizable or is particularly complex or clever, it may pass the initial patrol. Back up or reinforcements need to be called in. Through a "library" stored in the thymus gland, the immune system can check that it is not just an obscure hormone or part of the body. Then it can check if it is a known invader, and if so, has a reference on how to deal with it. If it is definitely an unknown invader, a full immune response is launched, manufacturing specific cells to kill it off. By this stage it is likely that you may have symptoms of infection. The infection will also try to get you to pass it on, by creating sneezing, which can travel at over 100 miles (160 km) per hour, coughing, which occurs at 60 miles (96.5 km) per hour, vomiting or diarrhea.

Generally, through the library of information stored about our body in the thymus gland, our immune system does not attack our friendly bacteria or own body cells. There are four hundred species of bacteria in the human colon that we rely on to help us digest our food. On some occasions the immune system may fail to recognize the body's own cells and the result is what is known as autoimmune disease. Autoimmune diseases include rheumatoid arthritis, celiac disease, diabetes mellitus type 1, systemic lupus erythematosus (SLE), or Sjögren's syndrome. This is where the immune system has gotten a bit confused and has turned on itself, the effects of which can be devastating.

Visceral Manipulation does not specifically address the immune system; rather, a practitioner will be looking for restrictions in the body shown by the General Listening. If the restrictions are affecting components of the immune system releasing these restrictions may enhance the function of these organs. However, this is not a primary focus in VM.

## Spleen

The spleen's immune functions are to store monocytes and to produce lymphocytes and antibodies—cells that help fight against infection. Monocytes are released into the bloodstream in the case of serious trauma to the body like a heart attack, gashing wound, or serious infection. The spleen also filters the blood to remove blood-borne parasites and aging blood cells. It works with red blood cells and iron levels in the blood. If a person cuts him- or herself, the spleen will release extra red blood cells to help the blood levels.

The spleen is not an essential organ for survival. It has been known to rupture in car accidents and then be removed, with the person leading a reasonably normal life after its removal. This is because the bone marrow and liver can double up to cover some of the spleen's functions, although it is suspected spleen removal will have an effect on immunity, and possibly life expectancy, in the long term.

The spleen is formed of lymphatic tissue and is the largest area of this tissue in the body. It is oval and measures about 5 inches (12 cm) in length 3 inches (7 cm) in width, being 1.5 inches (3 to 4 cm) deep. The average person's spleen weighs 20 to 22 ounces (170 to 180 g) at age twenty, but gradually decreases in weight throughout life. However, in certain conditions such as leukaemia, with glandular fever (mononucleosis) or malaria the spleen can increase in size to 11 to 15 pounds (5 to 7 kg)! It is situated on the left side of the body, tucked up under the diaphragm. (See Figure 14.1.) It has connections to the left kidney and the tail of the pancreas via a ligament. (See Figure 14.2.) The large intestine sits underneath the spleen and has a ligamentous attachment.

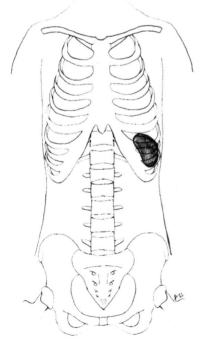

Figure 14.1. Spleen location

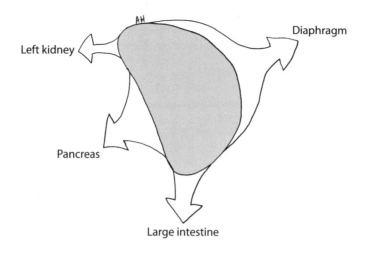

Figure 14.2. Spleen relations and attachments

Visceral Manipulation of the spleen has to be gentle because like the pancreas, it is a fragile organ. Treatment will often focus on ensuring the spleen has freedom to move in relation to its surrounding organs and tissues. For that reason treatment of the spleen may include the diaphragm, colon, left kidney, stomach, pancreas, and left lung. (See Figure 14.3.) Usually the spleen is entirely under the ribs, so if it is possible to feel it below this level it may be enlarged. Usually the patient will be lying on the right side, or possibly on the back for treatment of the spleen. Most of the treatment is likely to focus on Motility and on balancing this with either the Motility of the stomach or pancreas.

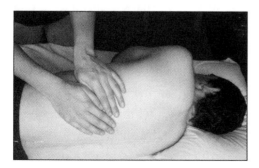

Figure 14.3. Spleen treatment

Possible causes of spleen issues:
- Immune system conditions or problems
- Childhood infections
- Cancer
- Vagus nerve problems
- Grief

Symptoms of spleen issues that may improve with VM:
- Intestinal issues in relation to digestion
- Anemia due to low iron levels
- Low back pain, left-sided, especially in children
- Lower rib cage pain, especially on the left
- Left-sided lower neck or shoulder pain
- Recurrent or frequent infections
- Grief, but being quite reserved with it

### A Frozen Shoulder

Heather came to me having met one of my other patients in the local supermarket. She had asked my patient if she could help her reach something off a shelf that was at shoulder height, as she had a frozen shoulder. This prompted my patient to give Heather my business card, as she had previously also had a frozen shoulder, with which I had helped her.

Using General Listening I felt Heather's body take me to the side and then down to her diaphragm level, closer to the back of the body. Using Local Listening I felt the attraction to her spleen. When I Listened to her spleen itself, it was apparent that there was a pull toward her stomach, probably along the gastrosplenic ligament. I asked Heather about her shoulder. She told me that her left one had started to hurt and become restricted about two years previously, shortly after the death of her husband. She had thought it was due to all the extra chores she had to do and the care she had given to him during his illness. She previously had some physiotherapy for it, but with only a little benefit. She found the therapy quite painful and so stopped attending.

Because Heather had come to me about her shoulder, I decided to assess the motion of her shoulders. I found that her left arm would only lift a third of its normal amount, both to the side and forward. When I applied Inhibition over the spleen, this motion increased to almost double its previous amount. This Mobility test confirmed my Listening that indicated the spleen was involved.

The next step was to find out more about the spleen restriction. Its associated restrictions were with the stomach, the phrenicocolic ligament, and the diaphragm. The spleen is supported by a sling called the phrenicocolic ligament. Phrenic means diaphragm and colic refers to colon, which are the two attachment sites for this ligament. Spleen restrictions can prevent the free downward movement of the diaphragm with breathing. This leads to mechanical tension in the tissues of the trunk and shoulder areas, which could account for Heather's symptoms. Additionally, the diaphragm and shoulder are both supplied by the phrenic nerve, so any binding in the area around the diaphragm can also be the underlying cause of shoulder restriction.

To provide greater ease of motion for the spleen, I brought Heather's spleen and stomach together in a direction of ease technique to encourage the tissues between them to regain their ease of motion and springiness. I then also brought the spleen and diaphragm toward one another to gently improve the slide and glide between them.

By the end of the appointment, Heather was amazed to find that despite my not having treated her shoulder, her movement had almost doubled and now was much more comfortable. I treated Heather seven times over the following months, and by the end of her sessions she had full use of her shoulder.

In Heather's case I have to wonder if her grief had added to her spleen tension, in addition to her change of workloads. Often frozen shoulders or shoulder pain are secondary to an internal organ restriction. While there are no hard and fast rules, the most common organs that refer to the shoulder area are the liver, gallbladder, stomach, and spleen. Additionally, the emotional connection with the spleen tends to be grief, which may have contributed to the issues in Heather's case.

# 15

# Nervous System

Jean-Pierre Barral, along with Alain Croibier, has developed an entire teaching curriculum dedicated to the peripheral nervous system. These are the nerves once they come out of the spinal column. This reflects the importance of the system, as it acts as the control mechanism for all body functions. It is like a huge telephone-wire network, linking up the brain to all parts of the body. Like organs, nerves need to be able to move properly in relation to their surrounding structures for normal function. Andrew Taylor Still, the developer of osteopathy, stated, "Every nerve must be free to act and do its part." (Quoted in Robert Ward's *Foundations for Osteopathic Medicine,* 2nd edition.) This shows how nerve Manipulation as developed by Barral and Croibier has followed its osteopathic principles. Due to the complexity of this system, and as this book is focused on Visceral Manipulation, only an overview of this work is included here.

Neural Manipulation (NM) is a branch of VM that aims to gently create movement and freedom within the peripheral nervous system. This is done by finding the points that are restricting the nerves, and their effects either on the other parts of that nerve or on the rest of the body. (See Figure 15.1.) When a nerve is fixed, it typically loses its ability to glide and/or stretch in length. The pressure both within and next to the nerve increases dramatically, and at the same time the tissues may change in consistency. This leads to the nerve having functional disturbances—rather like the electric wires during a storm. Nerve freedom of movement is essential for optimal blood and nerve supply going to the nerve. Nerve freedom of movement is also important for sending nerve impulses on. Additionally, NM aims to restore balance in the nervous system. For example, where there is a restriction in one arm, it may also affect the opposite arm. Allowing balance to return to the body can in turn affect the whole posture and nerve control of the body.

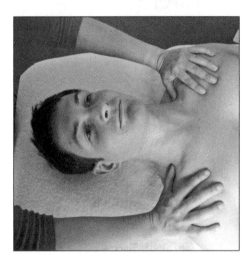

Figure 15.1. Checking nerve balance from one side to the other

Treatment to the nerves can be either on a nerve itself or on the surrounding structures to free up the nerve movement. Treatment to nerves is through precise applied pressure. Like blood vessels, nerves love to be elongated, so this often forms a part of the treatment. Additionally, the nerve branches often supply areas of skin, and these can be stimulated through such techniques as skin rolling to reflexively address deeper nerve issues. Treatment of the surrounding structures could involve the tissues the nerve supplies, perhaps an organ, fascia, blood vessel, or joint. Treatment can also include the structures that surround the nerve that are adding pressure onto the nerve. In a case like this there could be a spinal or cranial bone (that is, the bones in the head) restriction that affects the central nervous system (that is, the brain and spinal cord).

Also the nerve as it leaves the central nervous system through the openings in the vertebrae may be compressed by the vertebrae.

There may also be an emotional component in nerve restrictions. The VM techniques used for the tissues it supplies and for the emotional component are discussed in detail elsewhere in this book. As for all structures, the exact VM or NM treatment procedures used on the nervous system are determined by Listening to the body. Then throughout the treatment the practitioner will monitor how the patient's tissues are responding and modify his or her techniques accordingly. The goal of the VM practitioner is to be gentle and precise with the palpation, and to always think in three dimensions.

It is important to note that the release of nerve restrictions can have a favorable effect on the functioning of the corresponding visceral organs and muscles. Nerve control is involved in all body functions, and without it the organs and muscles would not function. Any changes in a nerve are processed by the brain. Therefore NM treatment of a nerve can affect not only the nerve itself, but all body tissues, via its connections to the rest of the nervous system through its relations to local tissues, through the fascial and postural connections throughout the body, and via its links to the organs, muscles, and skin it supplies.

Included here are a couple of cases that illustrate the potential effects of Neural Manipulation. The first one shows the effects NM can have on the visceral system, and the latter one a case of pain related to a nerve restriction.

### *Digestive Issues Due to Restricted Nerve Function*

Recently I met Lewis, who had a variety of symptoms including pain in the back of his head and around into his outer ear canal and jaw on the left. He had digestive dysfunction, a tendency to constipation, and a feeling of being stressed. He told me this started after some dental treatment about 6 months previously. On assessment, General Listening and cranial Local Listening took me to his left temporal bone (the bone on the side of the head that contains the ear canal).

When I listened to his temporal bone it was apparent that he had a restriction of the joint between the temporal bone and the occipital bone (the bone at the bottom/back part of the head). Additionally, his temporal bone had a compressed feel. I started off releasing his temporal bone, which almost immediately eased his pain in his head and jaw. Then I went on to release the suture (joint) between his temporal bone and occiput. (See Figure 15.2.) In this suture there is an opening called the jugular foramen, which is located in the bottom of the skull. This opening contains the jugular vein, which is responsible for eighty percent of the fluid drainage from the head and also holds several cranial nerves. One of the cranial nerves is the vagus nerve, which is responsible for the parasympathetic (or calming) nerve supply to much of the body. Restriction on this nerve seemed to be the mechanism that was causing his constipation, given that the vagus nerve governs peristaltic activity in the bowel.

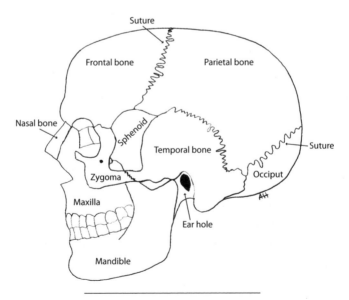

Figure 15.2. The skull and sutures

Once I had released the jugular foramen area, I then worked directly on the vagus nerve to insure it had freedom of movement. The word "vagus" comes from the Latin root for "vagrant," meaning "wanderer." This describes the nerve's long journey through the body to reach the abdominal organs. The vagus nerve runs through the chest area, where it travels along the esophagus (food pipe). It goes through the diaphragm to an area close to the stomach (known as the gastroesophageal junction) and supplies the digestive system. The most common sites of restriction for this nerve are as it leaves the skull at the jugular foramen and at the gastroesophageal junction.

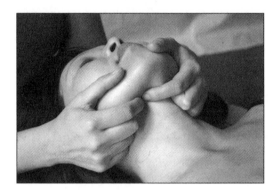

Figure 15.3. Treatment of a cranial nerve

Lewis' vagus nerve was also restricted at the gastro-esophageal junction. By placing my hand on his stomach I gently encouraged the downward glide of the esophagus as it transitioned through the diaphragm, which led to release of the gastroesophageal junction.

Lewis left the session feeling much improved in terms of head, ear, and jaw pain. He contacted me a few days later to tell me his bowel had normalized and his pain was virtually resolved.

### Highland Dancer's Foot Pain

In Scotland we have a style of dancing known as Scottish Highland Dancing. Many young people learn this, and there are regular competitions throughout the country each weekend at each town's Highland Games during the summer months. One of the most famous dances is the Highland Fling, which requires the dancer to leap from the right foot and land on the left at the start of the dance. When they are doing this leap in competitions, dancers have often been hanging around for some time waiting for their turn and so are not as warmed up as they would like to be. The result is that I have seen a number of teenaged girls with left foot pain from this dance injury.

The problem with each girl is more or less the same as Ailsa's. Ailsa was doing well—competing and getting a position in her age group most times. However, she began to experience pain in her foot, and she was not doing well at the competitions. She came to see me, and I observed that she was walking on the outer part of her foot. She had pain under her foot, and she had pain on pointing her toes. (Highland dancing involves point work, so this was a big problem for her).

I did General Listening, which took me to her left leg. I then Listened to the leg itself and found Listening attraction to the outer knee. This pulled down into the back of the calf and ankle. This followed the path of the posterior tibial nerve, so I started with the tibial nerve behind the knee. I found a restriction at this point, which I released, and then helped this area of the nerve elongate toward the foot. Then my Listening took me to the lower part of the leg at the ankle that the nerve has to go around on its journey into the foot, and there was another area of restriction. Once this was released I could treat the plantar nerves of the foot (the sole of the foot) where Ailsa was experiencing her symptoms. As I released these little nerves she suffered some pains across the sole of her foot and into the area that had been troubling her.

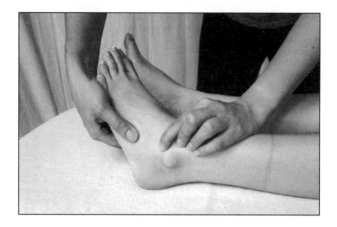

Figure 15.4. Treatment of a peripheral nerve in the foot

On her next visit Ailsa reported she had suffered significantly less pain. I treated her once again and agreed that she could restart her dancing (as I had advised rest to allow the nerve to recover on the previous visit—much to her dismay). I saw her two more times to support her as she returned to her dancing and competitions. She was able to dance for the rest of the season, although did come back into me with a slight recurrence following another poor landing, which we quickly resolved. Both she and her dance teacher sent a number of other dancers to me with very similar problems—a truly Scottish condition.

16

# The Emotions

Emotions play a huge role in our lives. When we feel an emotion, our body reacts. A person has only to think of a stressful situation for the jaw to clench, the shoulders to be raised up, and the muscles to tighten. Did you know it takes seventeen muscles to smile and forty-three to frown? Not surprisingly, the organs also react to emotions. Most people can remember feeling sick before going into an exam, having butterflies in their stomach when they were excited about something, having a heavy heart when they heard sad news, or finding it hard to breathe after they heard shocking news. Studies have been carried out that have found that listening to music is good for digestion and that epileptic patients who listen to Mozart's piano sonatas can dramatically decrease their chance of a seizure. It has also been medically proven that laughter is an effective painkiller. Likewise, when people have a physical problem they will simultaneously have an emotional reaction. Physical problems cause people pain and worry, or limits their daily activities and enjoyment. These problems result in the emotional changes people experience. Every restriction in the body has both a structural and emotional component; what varies is the percentage of each. What Visceral Manipulation can offer is to enhance health by addressing the physical component, which in turn helps to restore emotional balance.

Sometimes emotional responses last a few seconds or minutes and are relatively minor. Others are more severe or long lasting. These can really change the body's functioning and create physical problems. The symptoms of emotional reactions can be almost anything, with the more common ones being digestive spasms, heartburn, vomiting, fainting, ulcers, or more serious disease. Some organs react more quickly—for example, the gallbladder and stomach react to our everyday annoyances—while others are slower to react. All organs are connected to the brain physically and emotionally. At a July 2008 symposium in Jupiter, Florida, Barral stated, "The brain receives a combination of what is physical and emotional, and it doesn't make so much difference." This means that the brain is not able to clearly differentiate between physical and emotional messages, so for this reason emotions are an area that VM addresses, as otherwise many issues would not resolve.

So why do physical reactions come with emotions? This is a way for the brain and body to discharge psychological problems. The brain receives so much information that it cannot store it all—it can receive up to ten billion pieces of information per second. It then has to sift through all the information and sort out the most pressing pieces to deal with, discharging the rest so it is ready for the next onslaught in the following second. The organs act as discharge vessels for this extra information. When the stress is minor or short lived, a person may not be aware of this process and not experience any symptoms. However, when it is long lasting or more severe, he or she may start to experience symptoms. These symptoms serve to alert one to an issue that needs attending to, be it by making a change in one's life or expressing an emotion. In this way, a person may actually have a psychosomatic (mind-body) illness that is there to catch his or her attention and help the person to change. For further information on emotions and the body's response to them, see Jean-Pierre Barral's 2007 book, *Understanding the Messages of Your Body.* In this book, Barral states, "Thank goodness, we have psychosomatic reactions!" What we need to do is learn to listen to and understand these reactions.

Conversely, it may be that a physical reaction has led to an emotional issue. Feeling a small twinge in the low back may remind a person of being injured in a car accident one time. He or she may begin to remember how long and horrible the recovery process was at that time, and worry that it could happen again. This worry exacerbates the pain, and now the low back is excruciating. This leads to more worry, and the person decides to go to the emergency room. The result is that physical and emotional issues can become so intertwined that it often is hard to identify the initial trigger. Treating either component will help the person, but for full resolution to be achieved, both aspects need to be addressed.

Emotional responses are very individual. In a situation where someone is in a car with three others when they come to a railway crossing that is just closing, one person might be stressed by being held up because they are trying to get to the station to catch that train and now know they will miss it. One child could be scared of trains and so be upset at seeing one approaching. Another child's day might be made by having the opportunity to see the train pass. The factors that determine people's emotional responses are varied, and are linked to their previous experiences, general outlook on life, and state of health at the time.

## Visceral Manipulation and the Emotions

As in all VM sessions, the first step for the practitioner is to identify where to treat first. (See Chapter Five, "Visceral Manipulation Evaluation Techniques.") That there is an energy field around the body that can be photographed with Kirlian photography has been proven through scientific experiments. Most people have at some time been near someone and felt there was something strange about that person, or have known someone who made them feel good just by being around. What about the saying, "You could cut the tension in the room with a knife"? These are all experiences with people's energy fields. Emotions tend to express themselves by changes in this energy field. By using these factors the VM practitioner can pick up signals from the body about the emotional issues affecting a person at that moment. (See Figure 16.1.) Gail Wetzler, a teacher of VM and Director of the Visceral Manipulation Curriculum for the Barral Institute, during a 2007 class in New York told students, "When we touch an organ, we touch someone's mind."

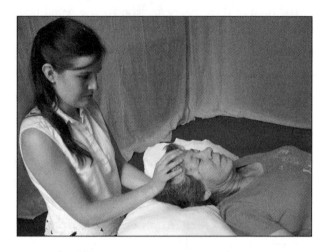

Figure 16.1. Working with the emotions

## Visceral Treatment for the Emotional Component

Treatment for the emotional component generally comes after treatment of the physical component. The emotional component may be stirred up when a particular area of the body is contacted, or the emotional issue may present initially. For example, if someone was hit in the jaw during an argument years ago, if the jaw is touched during a VM session, it may retrigger the emotional response of the anger at being hit.

There are centers in the brain that have been found to work with emotions. One of these centers is slightly to the right of midline on top of the head, and the others are on the forehead. They are connected to the limbic system, which is the system in the brain that deals with emotions. Visceral Manipulation practitioners work with these centers and their connections with the affected organ to open up processing possibilities for the body. (See Figure 16.2.) While feeling these connections the practitioner may find ways to increase the specificity of the treatment, such as feeling for how long the person has had the problem. Specifically identifying the trauma or the start of the issue allows the body to more fully resolve the problem. After the emotional and brain components have been treated, VM practitioners typically return to the affected organ and balance it to complete the session.

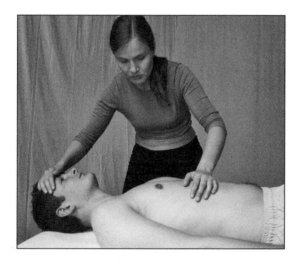

Figure 16.2. Treating the emotional component of a visceral issue

As a person's emotional and physical states are so intertwined, releasing the emotional component can lead to great physical improvement. Supporting someone to find a life's purpose, or see his or her situation in a different way, can totally alter that person's outlook and objectives.

## Emotions Related to Organs

With years of practice, Jean-Pierre Barral has found the following types of issues can be associated with individual organs.

Stomach (See Figure 16.3.)

- Social life
- Extroversion
- One's mission in life
- Appearances and the image one projects to others
- Problems with superiors
- Focus on the future
- Being excessively ambitious
- Acting seductively
- Fearing failure
- Flighty behavior
- Feeling powerful, in contrast with self-deprecation
- Spontaneous reactive anger
- Poor self-esteem
- Lack of confidence

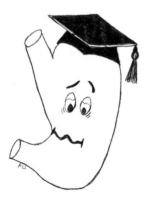

Figure 16.3. Stomach emotional expression— "Image we project to others with poor self-esteem underlying"

Duodenum, part of small intestine (See Figure 16.4)

- Dealing with one's true being
- Intolerance and frustration
- Insecurity
- Marked ambition

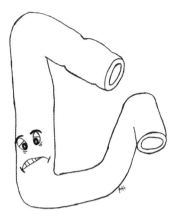

Figure 16.4. Duodenum emotional
expression—
"Frustration and intolerance"

Small and large intestines, most prone to psychosomatic reactions
- Great need to talk
- Faithful, meticulous, obstinate
- Great need for security and protection
- Tendency toward exaggeration and theatrics
- Hypochondriacal
- Need to be right and convince others
- Slightly obsessive
- Rigidity
- Great generosity
- Mood swings
- Hypersensitivity and tendency to paranoia

Liver (See Figure 16.5)
- Hard time knowing the self
- Dependency on the mother and the past
- Tendency toward pessimism and a fear of the future
- Lack of self-esteem, feeling insecure and hypersensitive
- Stuck in a routine
- Bad moods

- Lack of a fighting spirit
- Lack of creativity
- Anger
- Depression
- Phobias

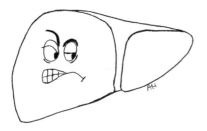

Figure 16.5. Liver emotional expression—
"Pessimism, bad moods, fits of anger, and depression"

Gallbladder (See Figure 16.6.)

- Material life is falling apart
- Worrying, constantly preoccupied and troubled
- Fear of conflict
- Extreme punctuality
- A need to stay in one place
- Finding it hard to deal with travel, departures, or separations
- Hypersensitivity or hyperactivity
- Fear of exams and confrontations
- Annoyance
- Slightly jealous

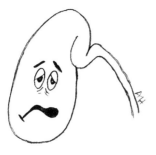

Figure 16.6. Gallbladder emotional expression—"Constant worry, feeling troubled, and annoyance"

Kidneys (See Figure 16.7.)

- Existential fear (deeply rooted)
- Depleted deep-seated energy reserves and lowered strength
- Fear and insecurity
- Need to lead
- Need to outdo oneself
- Deep-seated anger
- Generosity
- Cyclic pessimism

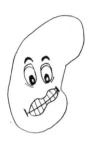 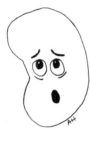

Figure 16.7. Kidneys emotional expression—"Non-identical twins dealing with fear and deep-seated anger"

Bladder (See Figure 16.8.)

- Importance of having control
- Emotional blackmail and guilt
- Obedience and submission
- Prudishness
- Shyness episodes

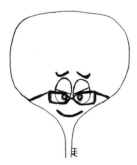

Figure 16.8. Bladder emotional expression— "A great need to keep control"

Lungs (See Figure 16.9.)

- Poor management of one's own territory
- Lack of self-confidence
- Lack of balance between "too much" and "not enough"
- Fear of being dominated
- Lack of authority
- Fear of suffocating or drowning
- Claustrophobia
- Fear of confrontation
- Withdrawal
- Fear of bothering people
- Dependency on others and a need for affection and attention
- Aggressiveness and hostility
- Helpfulness and generosity
- Suppressed feelings and childhood fears still present
- Rigidity
- Resignation to one's fate
- A vivid imagination

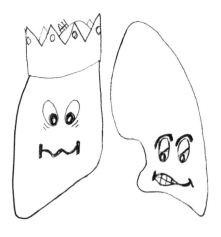

Figure 16.9. Lungs emotional expression—"Lack of balance between 'too much' and 'not enough,' fear, and withdrawal"

Heart (See Figure 16.10.)

- Need to be recognized, loved, and liked; fear of not being loved
- Excessive attachment to others
- Love given and received in one's life
- Fear of being abandoned
- Jealousy
- Distrust
- Fear of being judged
- Generosity
- Need to be flattered and rewarded
- Stage fright
- Fear in general
- Guilt or hatred
- Pain of severe loss
- Too powerful an emotion
- Distress
- Joy and happiness

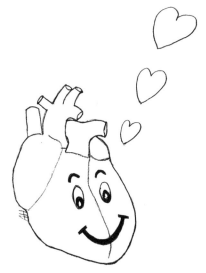

Figure 16.10. Heart emotional expression—"The love you give in your life"

Breasts
- Recognizing femininity
- Submissive
- Need to protect and be protected
- Need for emotional security
- Shyness
- Motherly love
- Loneliness, whether real or imaginary
- Difficulty dealing with life transitions or breakups in relation-ships
- Unfulfilled wish to have a child
- Feelings of guilt or failure
- Submission and fatalism
- Difficulty finding one's place or role in life
- Hiding feelings behind a façade of serenity

Genital organs (See Figure 16.11.)
- One's origin and future
- Total protection one needs in life
- Need for a shelter
- Need to receive and give
- Fear of being abandoned
- Fear of not doing well, or of being judged
- Fear of expressing things

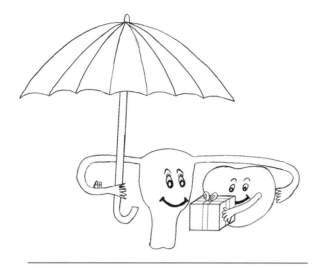

Figure 16.11. Genital organs emotional expression—
"A need for shelter and a need to give and receive"

Pancreas (See Figure 16.12.)

- Grief
- Something difficult for one to accept
- Death of a child
- Unbearable stress
- Serious illness
- Meeting one's own mortality
- An unsatisfying life
- Severe childhood trauma

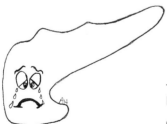

Figure 16.12. Pancreas emotional
expression—"Grief"

Spleen

- Reacting to serious events that can upset a person for life
- Absorption of the most severe shocks
- Pessimism
- Deep sadness
- Unaccepted deaths
- Despair and inconsolable sorrow
- Severe childhood trauma

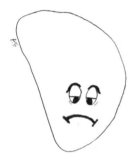

Figure 16.13. Spleen emotional expression—"Deep sadness"

Due to the interrelation of physical and emotional issues, and the similarities in symptoms between the two, it is imperative that both elements are addressed when present. For example, a stomach ulcer that has been triggered by stress has just as much of a physical symptom as the results of a mechanical trauma such as an accident. If the emotional component is not addressed, often the physical symptoms will remain or recur, hence the importance of this part of the VM approach to help the body find its pathway to health.

### An Emotional Cause of Low Back Pain

Eilidh was a forty-one-year-old woman who came to me with her low back pain. She had been to various therapists, and I was her last resort. When I first met Eilidh she told me about her career and her travels, and how they were affected by this ongoing low back pain.

When I placed my hand on her head for General Listening, Eilidh's body tilted forward to the point where she almost fell off her feet. The premise of General Listening is that the body "hugs the problem"—and falling forward indicates that the body is going toward the emotional-electromagnetic field. This is where the body is at the limit of compensation and wants help and attention first.

Manual Thermal Evaluation highlighted Eilidh's left kidney and uterus, the organs that were involved in the Emotional Listening. I began the treatment by mobilizing Eilidh's left kidney, and then used a direction of ease technique on the line of tension between her left kidney and uterus. Then I moved to her head and helped to wake up the connection between her brain and the left kidney.

As we were working, a couple of tears rolled down Eilidh's cheek. She told me that she was not sure why she was crying, only that she felt so sad that she might not have children due to her age and lack of a partner. This was something that bothered her on and off and for some reason had just popped into her mind as I was treating her. I explained to her that by helping her body find the connections with the emotional components of her physical symptoms, it might bring up conscious awareness of the issue. This conscious awareness could assist in resolving her physical pain.

I saw Eilidh three weeks later. She told me that her back had twinged a few times in the days after her last treatment, but then she had been pain free for more than two weeks. She also thought about her concerns over having children and resolved that she would only have children if she met the right partner. She certainly did not want to become a single parent and recognized she was happy to remain childless if the right partner did not come along. Did she gain this insight and clarity about her emotional issue as a result of releasing her tissues? Or did her tissues release through her exploration and resolution of the emotional issues? Perhaps a bit of both.

## *An Emotional Component of a Physical Problem*

Maisie was a fourteen-year-old girl, who came to me because she was unable to eat due to severe abdominal pain and cramping that was brought on by food. Gradually she become more scared of bringing the pain on, and so did not want to eat. Her weight dropped as low as 70 pounds (32 kg), and she was tube fed at times. As a result she was unable to attend school.

Initially her treatment was to address the issue of her digestive system, starting with the stomach, duodenum, and sphincters to restore Mobility and Motility and allow peristalsis to work effectively again. However, Maisie did not gain weight. Her mother told me that because of her fear of bringing on the pain Maisie still would not eat much. In addition, she was losing contact with her school and worried about her studies. Overall it is no surprise she had developed an emotional reaction that was now holding her back from recovering from her physical state.

I treated Maisie to help reestablish the connections and patterning from her emotional centers in her brain to her stomach. She commented that she felt less worried and more relaxed by the end of the session. When I next saw her she had worked out a system of rewards for weight gain with her mother and generally seemed much more upbeat. She was increasing her portion sizes, and gradually over the months that followed started to regain some of her lost pounds. She also enjoyed the rewards that she received as each weight target was achieved.

# 17

# Additional Thoughts on How Visceral Manipulation Can Help

Visceral Manipulation is used to locate and treat restrictions throughout the body. It encourages a person's own natural self-healing mechanisms to improve the functioning of the organs, counteract the negative effects of stress, allow movement throughout the body, release pain, and positively influence general metabolism and health. Throughout this book each system has been discussed in detail and each section contains a list of conditions that VM may help. As can be gathered from this, through its holistic approach, VM has an incredibly wide scope. Below is discussion about conditions that relate to specific age groups—for instance, children. However, it is important to remember that a person does not actually have to suffer any symptoms for his or her body to benefit from treatment. As the saying goes, "An ounce of prevention is worth a pound of cure." Additionally, any symptom can be due to a wide variety of causes. For this reason one does not have to be suffering from symptoms related to organ dysfunction for the organs to be treated. Conversely, someone may have symptoms related to an organ and find that the practitioner treats an area that seems to that person to be unrelated.

## Organ Displacements

Contrary to popular belief, it is actually quite unusual for an organ to be displaced. For example, kidneys can drop by a few centimeters (called ptosis), which can be seen on scans and can lead to kidney infections, stones, and tiredness, but most organs are so well held in position they can not become displaced unless there has been major surgery. In most cases problems arise because organs lose their full natural range of movement. As most scans are done in a stationary position, they are very good at showing organ position but in many cases somewhat less effective at revealing organ Mobility dysfunction.

## Organ Removal and Visceral Manipulation

When an organ has been surgically removed, the body will have various issues to deal with. There is the scarring from the surgery itself and the adaptations the body has to make to cope without that organ. The body may pass functions over to other organs that the removed organ used to perform. There is an empty space left by the organ's removal. The other organs will expand and drop into this space due to the altered pressure and support dynamics. For example, a woman who has a hysterectomy often has a slight dropping of her other organs up to and including her kidneys, as they all move into the space where her uterus had been. In addition, the initial cause of the organ dysfunction may have been outside the organ, physically, chemically, or emotionally, and thus the underlying cause was not treated by the surgery. For example, even after a gallbladder full of gallstones has been removed, the rest of the body can very much benefit from VM sessions. This will help the body balance and resolve the possible digestive dysfunction that may have contributed a back pressure on the gallbladder and caused it to clog up in the first place.

## Organ Transplants

Organ transplants are becoming more common. They are a lifesaver in many cases. Visceral Manipulation can definitely benefit the person who has had a transplant, although the techniques used will be modified. When an organ is transplanted it is not necessarily connected in exactly the same way as the original one was. Perhaps the original one had been diseased, and created some additional changes in the tissues surrounding it. For this reason, as a practitioner may not know exactly how an organ is connected, or how its blood or nerve supply is functioning, he or she will only use Motility techniques on the transplanted organ itself, rather than risking that Mobility techniques that might displace or disrupt anything. The practitioner may balance it with other surrounding organs to allow it to function in better harmony with the body.

## Can Visceral Manipulation Deal with Major Disease, or Just Minor Problems?

I always state that VM can work with almost any problem, any stage, and any age. But as discussed in the healthcare overview chapter, Chapter Three, I see VM as fitting into complementary therapy. That means that it complements other medical care. While VM may help with most conditions, it is not per se intended to be a lifesaver or preserver. Visceral Manipulation is mainly effective in the realm of the chronic rather than the acute condition. When major, potentially terminal conditions are involved, it can be used as an adjunct to other medical care.

## Whom It Can Help—Age Groups and Life Stages

Visceral Manipulation is useful for all age groups, from tiny babies to the elderly. There are some modifications made for different stages of life.

Jean-Pierre Barral teaches: "We adapt the manipulation accordingly and adjust the hand pressure with respect to the type of patient." (Quoted in a John Weiler article posted on the Barral Institute website, at www.barralinstitute.com.)

In babies and children who cannot crawl or roll over themselves, only Motility techniques are used, as opposed to any Mobility. (See Figure 17.1.) This is because at this stage, the fragility of the developing tissues makes a gentler approach preferable. Likewise this approach is used with the very frail, or women who are pregnant or breastfeeding. All these groups have less stability in their tissues.

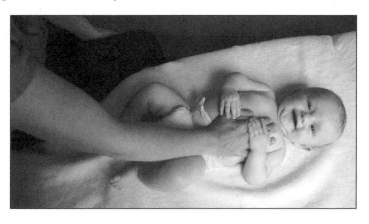

Figure 17.1. Baby receiving Visceral Manipulation

Jean-Pierre Barral reports that he often uses VM with children, and that the liver and kidneys can be particularly indicated, due to the infections, digestive, and waterworks issues with which children frequently have to cope. Additionally, he suggests that treatment on the head and of the digestive system is beneficial. While these are his comments on treating children, first an evaluation of their health will be made. Then the practitioner will treat as appropriate for the child's age, developmental stage, and condition, and according to the Listening findings the practitioner receives.

Some of the more frequent issues experienced by children and babies that may be helped by Visceral Manipulation treatment are:

- Constipation and gastritis
- Persistent vomiting
- Vesicoureteral reflux
- Infant colic

Pregnancy puts a particular strain on the body. As the uterus expands to as much as one thousand times its prepregnancy size it forces the repositioning of many other organs, including the entire digestive system, the bladder, and the liver. It can even affect the lungs and heart. If any one of these organs has a restriction in it, movement may well be emphasized and cause symptoms as the fetus grows. Additionally, the blood vessels and nerves may become restricted, and pressure changes throughout the body are inevitable. Pregnant women store up to 7 quarts (8 l) of extra fluid in the body and will gain about 25 pounds (13 kg, or nearly 2 stone) in weight. (See Figure 17.2.) Her body has to not only supply her needs but also meet the needs of her growing baby, meaning her digestive, immune, breathing, circulatory, and waterworks systems all have to work extra hard to meet these demands. For these reasons, while strong pressure on the abdomen is avoided, treatment may be very beneficial to aid fluid flow, digestion, and general well-being for the pregnancy.

## Are There Any Contraindications?

With VM there are very few total contraindications to treatment; however, there are various contraindications for certain techniques on different ages or conditions, which have been outlined as we have gone through the body. In general, Motility techniques and sphincters are never contraindicated. These techniques are safe to use with all people.

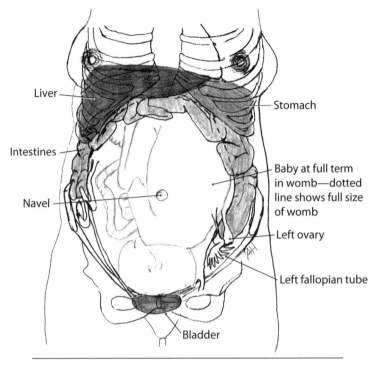

Liver

Stomach

Intestines

Baby at full term
in womb—dotted
line shows full size
of womb

Navel

Left ovary

Left fallopian tube

Bladder

Figure 17.2. The effect of pregnancy on the internal organs

Practitioners are taught to act cautiously, and so may choose not to treat someone if they have cause for concern. Specifically, a practitioner will be looking for signs of serious disease that might be either life threatening or could deteriorate if not attended to immediately. If they find something of concern, they will refer the patient to a doctor for further assessment. This may be, for example, a tumor, a bleed in part of the body, a thrombosis, a perforated ulcer, enlarged lymph nodes, unexplained weight loss, aneurism, a heart condition, or an infection. When working in the pelvis if there is suspected pregnancy or an intrauterine device (IUD), treatment may not be appropriate at that time. However, each case is individual, and as long as practitioners are aware of any possible circumstances that might mean there is a contraindication for

VM, they will judge all cases on their merits and the parts of the body that need treatment.

If a practitioner finds that there are signs of an acute infection, inflammation, or recent trauma it is best to allow the body to deal with the current issue rather than giving it more changes to cope with. Applied during a crisis, VM could overload the body with information. After the crisis has passed, VM can be very useful in helping the body reassess the adaptations it made to cope at the time of the crisis. This can prevent residual compensations that might lead to restrictions or further problems down the line. This is rather like the effects of adverse weather conditions on a community, for example a hurricane. During the storm everyone copes the best they can, with their windows boarded up, relying on stored provisions and evacuating or sheltering from the weather. After the storm has passed, slowly life can return to normal. Some adaptations have to be made, such as living elsewhere for a time to allow repair to storm damage. With help normal life can resume once this period of recovery is complete, as long as the assistance required has been available.

## Treatment Times and Regularity— How Much Treatment Will Be Needed?

At the initial consultation, practitioners should be able to give an idea of how often and for how long they will need to see someone. This will depend on the person's condition, pathway to health, and goals for treatment. In general, Jean-Pierre Barral suggests most people will notice change in three to five sessions, although in some very long-term or severe problems, it may be longer than this. Some problems will change rapidly and others more gradually depending on the condition, how long someone has had it, and how the body responds. All people are individuals, and every person is different.

Depending on the condition, the frequency of visits will be determined—the average is typically around one visit every two to three weeks. This allows the tissues time to adjust between appointments. However, this treatment schedule could be much shorter, say, twice a week, or up to once every six to eight weeks, depending on the individual. Sessions also vary in length according to the practitioner's style and the patient's needs. Sessions could be as short as ten minutes, perhaps with a baby, up to an hour or more in some cases. This is something to discuss with the practitioner and depends on how the body responds to treatment.

In VM the purpose is to help inform the body so it can heal itself. Therefore it should be a partnership between the patient and the therapist to allow for maximum healing. This is the reason that a practitioner may suggest leaving several weeks between appointments to allow the body time to self-correct in response to the changes that have been made during a treatment session. The patient may also receive recommendations of dietary, lifestyle or mental changes that can be made to allow the body to recover more fully. A patient must remember that he or she has a lot more time between therapy sessions than in them, so how the body is treated during this time can make a huge impact on that person's health.

Depending on the issue, appointments may have to be very precisely scheduled. For example it is not as effective to treat a woman during the first days of her menstrual cycle. However, in some instances if her symptoms are pain or cramping, at that time, it may be advisable for her practitioner to feel her body at that point in her cycle to evaluate the tissue tension during menstruation. Appointments may be scheduled at a time of day when a baby has its colic episode or during the particular phase of digestion when someone experiences digestive discomfort.

In general, Visceral Manipulation aims to remove restrictions in the body, allowing it to return to optimal functioning. In many cases once the restrictions have been resolved there is no need for ongoing care. If the appropriate primary cause has been treated and there are no lifestyle issues that cause the problem to return, there is no reason why it should recur. However, in some situations ongoing treatment may be indicated. For example there may be various compensatory changes the body has had to make to cope with the restriction and these may or may not be able to fully self-release. Also, people are not designed to sit at a computer, drive, or perform repetitive tasks all day. In cases where there has been structural change through surgery, accident, or illness, some ongoing care may be of benefit. These are all points for the patient to discuss with the practitioner.

In some cases it may be that VM is not going to help a condition. The practitioner may know this in advance, or it may be that the patient is not responding as it was hoped to treatment. If either the patient or the practitioner feels that the relationship is not working or the treatment is not helping as much as it could, then the practitioner may be able to make further recommendations as to the next step for effective health-care. In my experience, about eighty percent of my patients do benefit from treatment, with the rest either having an issue that requires referral to another healthcare professional or simply not responding to treatment. I remember at one point feeling frustrated that a particular patient was not recovering as I had hoped and discussing that patient's case with a colleague, who replied, "Alison, if you could help everyone you would be a saint!" A good lesson for every practitioner to remember.

## What If It Seems Like a Condition Is Very Long Term, or Symptoms Change, Plateau, or Relapse over the Course of Treatment?

Many patients I see have been everywhere else first and come to me as a last resort. This is probably due to the relative lack of familiarity with VM, along with few practitioners, certainly in Scotland where I work. This means most of my patients are coming to me with longer standing conditions or injuries. Recent traumas and conditions are usually faster to adapt and heal, but old injuries and compensations may also be relieved over a number of sessions. The joy of VM is that it is able to address conditions that have compensations and several layers or factors contributing to them in an efficient and orderly manner.

However, when there has been a problem for years and many compensations have developed, it may be that longer-term treatment is required. The catch in this is that neither the patient nor the practitioner needs to become despondent, but rather they should monitor progress, noting even smaller changes in the patient's body and seeing them as steps along the way. It is not uncommon for symptoms to change before they get better, as tissues work out their tensions with the changes made during treatment sessions. Likewise, it is also possible that a patient will suffer relapses or have times where improvement seems to have plateaued. These times can be emotionally upsetting but are natural steps along the way, as body tissues can only adapt so far and so fast, and may fatigue easily or still be prone to infection or the effects of diet, exercise, allergies, or emotions. It is best for a patient to discuss any of these issues with his or her practitioner as they occur rather than abandoning treatment and perhaps being deprived of the full benefits that VM may give. Usually after a period of plateau or relapse in a condition, progress is often quicker and recovery easier than they were initially.

## Are the Changes Permanent, or Does One Have to Keep Returning for More?

With VM, a major part of any session is identifying through the General and Local Listening where the main restriction is in the body on any given day. The approach is aimed at discovering which restrictions are having the greatest influence on a body at the time of the appointment. This is the area that the practitioner will then treat. The reason this is so important is that if the practitioner treats the primary area of restriction, it will often lead to resolution of other restrictions and compensations. This means that VM changes are long lasting.

However, that is the simplistic part of the story. As many problems people have are long standing or very severe, it may not be possible to fully address an issue in one session, and I do not want to mislead you to think this would be the case. For example, if someone has some scar tissue that has been there for twenty years, it is unlikely that the problem will be resolved in one session. In the twenty years there will be many ways a body has found to work around this area of adhesion. After the first session the patient's body needs time to respond and find how it is going to function with the change VM creates to the dry, tethered area. Additionally, there may be many layers to the scar, not just a physical restriction but possibly blood or nerve flow disruptions to the area, or an emotional component related to the original injury. These areas may also need to be treated to allow resolution and permanent change. The pathway to health is very individual.

## Are There Any Side Effects?

Visceral Manipulation is an incredibly safe therapy. To say there are no side effects would not be entirely correct, but the side effects are minor, such as perhaps aches in the days after treatment as the body is adapting to the changes. Mild nausea, a slight headache or fuzziness, bloating, tiredness, or changes in bowel or bladder function are all possible.

## Can I Help Myself?

Absolutely. Indeed, in Barral's excellent book *Understanding the Message of Your Body* (2007), he suggests, "First of all, do everything you can to stay healthy." This means that paying attention to your diet, exercise, and relaxation regime, avoiding unnecessary toxins, managing your stress levels, and understanding your emotions will not only help you heal from disease but also help prevent future problems. If you have symptoms already, see these as an opportunity. Instead of running to the pharmacist and picking up some painkillers for the headache you woke up with this morning, why not spend a few minutes thinking over what you did yesterday. Did you drink and eat enough of the appropriate things, did you get a good balance of fresh air and exercise, and how were your stress levels? If you can identify the triggers of your issue then you are on the first step to preventing the problem recurring. You may even be able to alleviate your headache by correcting the issue that created it—for example drinking more water or managing your stress levels. This then means you have learned from the experience, and it can become a positive contribution to your future health. *Understanding the Messages of Your Body* can help you in starting to listen to your own body.

# 18

# Practitioners of Visceral Manipulation

Visceral Manipulation is generally undertaken as a postgraduate study. It is now included in some European osteopathic training, but otherwise is an additional therapy that all manual therapy practitioners may add to their repertoire. The requirements to train in Visceral Manipulation are simply to have a qualification or license in some form of healthcare whereby you are able to apply manual therapy to the body, and an interest in anatomy. Jean-Pierre Barral has decided to open his work up to a variety of practitioners from different disciplines, which means VM can be more widely available and help more patients.

Most commonly practitioners will be osteopaths, medical doctors, chiropractors, doctors of traditional Chinese medicine, naturopathic physicians, physiotherapists, occupational therapists, shiatsu therapists, massage therapists, or Rolfers, although this list is by no means exclusive.

Training in Visceral Manipulation is currently modular. The classes are organized through the Barral Institute. Training programs have been running for twenty-five years. Classes are organized worldwide, and a list of all countries offering training is available. Teachers of VM all are active practitioners, working in clinical practice. They have trained extensively in the techniques and then been through a program of repeating classes, assisting classes and, finally, an apprentice program before being certified to instruct; this assures high-quality instructors and standards of training. For further information on training, see www.barralinstitute.com.

## How to Find a Practitioner

As with any therapy, it is essential that people find a practitioner with whom they feel comfortable. The Barral Institute (www.barralinstitute.com) has a list of practitioners that have trained with them. In general, people who have completed more classes are likely to have more skills. It is a good idea to contact the clinic where the practitioner works, enquire how much he or she uses VM, and whether the practitioner is able to work with your specific concerns. If it sounds like the practitioner will be able to work with your issues, you should see whether you feel comfortable and able to work with the practitioner to get the help required. Often we hear of new therapies or practitioners through word of mouth from their satisfied patients. Of course, personal recommendation is always a good line to follow.

To summarize, these are the points to look for when choosing a VM practitioner:

- Do they have the training? This can be easily checked by consulting www.barralinstitute.com and clicking on "Find a Therapist" or by contacting a local branch of the Barral Institute.

- Contact the practitioner and check if they work with your type of condition with VM.

- Talk to your friends locally and see if they can recommend a practitioner to you.

- Meet the practitioner. If you do not feel comfortable with them in any way, you may want to look for another practitioner with whom you do feel comfortable.

- Ask questions—your practitioner may not realize you are unclear about either something concerning your condition or about how VM functions.

- If you are not getting the desired results, discuss this with your practitioner. He or she may be able to make suggestions about what else you can do at home to assist the process. Your practitioner may also be able to help you with your expectations and understanding of how VM is working with you. Being an educated, proactive partner in your healthcare will ensure you achieve optimum results with any type of treatment.

- Remember, just because you have consulted one therapist, you do not belong to them. You are free to go elsewhere or leave treatment if that feels right to you. Just be sure you are making an educated decision.

- Trust your gut feeling—if it doesn't feel right then it probably isn't!

### Fergus Needed Someone He Felt Confident In

The story of Fergus is an example of someone needing to feel comfortable with a practitioner. Fergus was a sixty-five-year-old man who came to see me for his low back pain. On initial meeting he asked me if I had any training. I told him of my training and my experience. He said that the problem was that he just felt that I looked too young for him to have any confidence in me, and while even though I had been recommended to him by a friend, he just felt he could not take me seriously. For that reason we decided that he would go and find another practitioner, as we both agreed that if he felt so strongly about this he was not going to take any suggestions or treatment I offered seriously. This might therefore inhibit him from any potential benefit. Unfortunately, that was about five years ago, and I now mourn that my looks no longer cause the same dilemma for patients!

## Worldview

Visceral Manipulation is rapidly spreading around the globe. The Barral Institute currently teaches classes on all continents except Antarctica. While classes are not available in every country, practitioners do travel for training and VM is becoming more widespread.

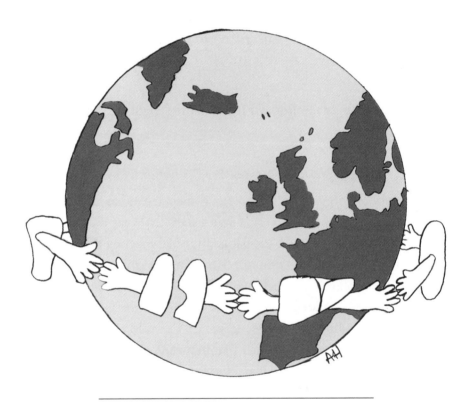

Figure 18.1. Visceral Manipulation around the globe

19

# Research

The following information is provided as a summary of some of the research involving Visceral Manipulation and Neural Manipulation. All the sources are listed in full in the "References" section of this book if you wish to read more details about these subjects. Additional resources can be found at www.barralinstitute.com.

## Imaging Motility

John-Pierre Barral and Pierre Mercier, DO, along with the help of radiologist Serge Cohen, MD, used intravenous pyelography to visualize the passage of a dye through the kidneys. They were able to see that even with the breath held, the kidneys continued to move repeatedly 1.5 inches (3 cm) vertically and laterally. This clearly indicated that the organs do have an intrinsic motion.

## Evidence of Organ Movement with Breathing

In a three-year study, Georges Finet and Christian Williame used X-rays and echograms and then videotaped them to look at how the organs move with breathing. This duplicated and confirmed similar studies performed by Barral in the early 1980s. When a person breathes the diaphragm moves up and down. With this diaphragmatic motion and the imaging, Finet and Williame were able to show that the organs under the diaphragm (stomach, liver, pancreas, kidney, duodenum, and intestines) move on response to the downward pressure of the diaphragm on an in-breath, and rise higher in the body in response to the diaphragmatic attraction on an out breath.

They went on to consider how abnormalities such as constipation or stomach disorders affected this motion. Their conclusion in every case was that an abnormality would either increase or reduce the movement of that organ; for example, in diarrhea the intestines gained extra movement, while with constipation they decreased in motion. Additionally, Finet and Williame considered how the organs moved in relation to one another. They found that various organs moved in the same way as one another, confirming once again the theory that dysfunction of one organ could lead to dysfunction of others through its altered motion.

They mapped the reproducible patterns of movement the organs have in a resting position. For example, they noted that the fundus of the stomach (top part) descends by 1.15 inches (29 mm), moves forward by slightly more than 1 inch (20 mm), and to the right by just under 0.2 inch (6 mm). They repeated this for each part of the liver, kidneys, spleen, stomach, duodenum, and small intestine, which also has reproducible movement patterns.

## Clinical Implications
## of Adhesions Following Surgery

Michael Diamond and Michael Freeman state that adhesions (e.g., infections, chemical irritation, surgery, or endometriosis, all of which disrupt the peritoneum and produce inflammation) remain a clinically relevant problem, and in nearly every compartment in the body. They report, "adhesions are prevalent in all surgical fields, which can lead to impaired organ functioning, decreased fertility, bowel obstruction, difficult re-operation, and possibly pain. Even when lysed, adhesions have a great propensity to reform."

## Adhesions and How They Affect the Body

Marcel Binnebosel, Uwe Klinge, Raphael Rosch, Karsten Junge, Petra Lynen-Jansen, and Volker Schumpelick collected tissue samples from forty patients. Tissue samples were evaluated using cross-polarization microscopy by two independent blinded observers. The adhesions ranged from half a month to twenty years old. All the patients had undergone previous abdominal surgery, some of them repeated times. The findings revealed that "even in mature surgical adhesions the distinct cellular components as well as the extra-cellular matrix proteins may reflect an interactive cross-talk between adhesion and stroma-derived cells as a consequence of a permanent process of disturbed remodelling." From this it has been concluded that adhesions lead to a risk of developing complications such as small bowel obstruction, chronic abdominal pain, and infertility in women.

## Visceral Manipulation for Low-Back Spinal Dysfunction

Gail Wetzler studied the effects of Visceral Manipulation on low back pain in thirty patients who consulted her between 1989 and 1991. Some of the patients had received previous manual therapy treatment, but not VM. On average, they had six to seven treatments each of VM. Evaluation using VM techniques pointed to the involvement of various organs as causes of the low back pain. The most common organs were the large and small intestines, which were involved with more than ninety-six percent and eighty-five percent of patients, respectively. The uterus, kidney, duodenum, and liver were the next most commonly involved organs. Results were measured via a pain scale that the patients completed, neurological testing, and movement and strength tests of the low back. The results showed marked improvement in all but two of the cases across all tests, leading to the conclusion that "low back spinal dysfunction may be more effectively and efficiently resolved with the addition of Visceral Manipulation into the treatment program."

## Fluoroscopy on Common Bile Duct

In 1980 Jean-Pierre Barral performed experiments using fluoroscopy to image the common bile duct, which is the tube from the gallbladder to the digestive system. He found that stretching the common bile duct increased the passage of bile from the gallbladder.

## Visceral Manipulation for Dyspepsia

Mary Harrow carried out a study on the effectiveness of Visceral Manipulation for dyspepsia. Dyspepsia, also known as gastroesophageal reflux, leads to the symptom of heartburn and is a common complaint. This case studied the use of VM on the gastroesophageal junction, that is, the region where the stomach and esophagus (food pipe from the mouth) join, on five patients. Harrow's findings were that after one manipulation of the gastro-oesophageal junction the symptoms in four of the five patients reduced significantly and the episodes happened less frequently. However, Barral recommends that treatment be repeated and that other associated areas be treated. Further treatment was not done in this study, so perhaps the effectiveness of treatment for dyspepsia is actually higher.

This study has not been published but was carried out through the Colorado Springs Osteopathic Foundation: Center for Osteopathic Education and Research, Colorado Springs Osteopathic Foundation, Colorado Springs, Colorado.

## Effects of Visceral Treatment on Digestive Abnormalities in Children with Autistic Disorders

Ioná Bramati Castellarin and Margit Janossa studied thirteen children between three and eight years of age who were given one session per week for five weeks of abdominal Visceral Manipulation. The children's parents filled in a questionnaire before and after treatment, which formed the material for the study. Statistical analysis of the results showed significant improvement in the children's symptoms of bloating, diarrhea, constipation, and abdominal pain. There were also improvements in social communication, including in respect to "lack of awareness of social rules, poor comprehension of verbal instructions, and cannot make friends."

## Effects of an Approach Including Visceral Treatment on Children with Poor Bladder Control

Diane R. Nemett, Barbara A. Fivush, Ranjiv Mathews, Nathalie Camirand, Marlo A. Eldridge, Kathy Finney, and Arlene C. Gerson found improvement in bladder control in twenty-one children when they received manual therapy including cranial, dural, visceral, vascular, and lymphatic treatments. This was compared with using "standard treatments," which included medications, establishment of timed voiding and evacuation schedules, dietary modifications, behavior modifications, pelvic floor retraining, biofeedback training, and treatment of constipation. The study concluded the improvement in dysfunctional urination was due to several factors, including improvement in normal alignment and Mobility. Treatment outcomes were measured by portable bladder ultrasound or an X-ray procedure. Furthermore, they found that there were no side effects, and in all cases treatment improved postural alignment and flexibility.

## Fluoroscopy on Ureter

In 1986 Scali and Giraud performed fluoroscopy imaging on the ureters, that is, the tubes from the kidneys to the bladder. They found that the efficiency of the ureters was increased by forty percent by stretching them.

## Lung Disease Studies

In Grenoble, France, Barral studied the effects of lung disease on the motions in the chest cavity. He was able to study patients when they were opened up for surgery, or in some cases, study them at post mortems. He found that the directions of movements and the pressures of the lungs changed with disease, and that these changes altered the axes of motion for all the supporting structures including the bones and muscles. He also found that these changes affect the digestive system, the heart, neck, and so on. In the end he was able to observe and feel how the whole body becomes involved. These changes were visible through changes in tissue structure, where some tissues had become thickened or lost their elasticity. This showed how visceral changes can significantly affect other systems and structures and over time lead to muscular or skeletal change and symptoms. Additionally, Barral was able to observe how a relatively minor lung injury could be responsible for considerable disease and disturbance. And he was also able to observe the effects of time on a minor organ problem and how far-reaching it could become if left untreated.

## Kidney Study with Ultrasound

Jacques-Marie Michallet used ultrasound to study the effects of Visceral Manipulation on the kidneys. He selected twenty-five patients with renal ptosis (kidney dropped lower from its normal position). Following manipulation, in every case the kidney was immediately able to move farther (on average by 0.75 inch, or 17.2 mm) when scanned by ultrasound. He then asked the patients to return two months later and found that in the cases he rescanned, they had gained an extra 0.25 inch (8.6 mm) of movement on average, meaning a total gain of 1 inch (28.5 mm). This study demonstrates the need to give the body time to change itself between sessions, and demonstrates the power of the body to self-heal between treatments. It also shows that with VM it is possible to affect the amount of movement of an organ substantially and accurately even though, as in the case of the kidney, it lies very deep in the body and is not easy to feel. Additionally, Michallet notes that the distance the kidney moved was directly in proportion to the person's size, which is logical, so in one case the kidney actually moved 2 inches (55 mm) with manipulation.

## Doppler on Arterial Blood Circulation

In 1982, Barral and Louis Rommeveaux, with the help of Bernard Morzol carried out experiments on the effect of Visceral Manipulations on the radial and vertebral basilar arteries using a Doppler machine to measure blood flow. They found without any doubt that immediate improvement or restoration of blood flow was possible following slight manipulation of an abdominal organ.

More recently, Barral and Alain Croibier have carried out further studies on three hundred to four hundred people showing the effects of Visceral Manipulation and Nerve Manipulation of an artery on blood flow. They did this by measuring the flow with a Doppler machine before and after the arterial manipulation, finding a significant improvement in arterial flow was possible.

## Fallopian Tube Treatment Study

As reported in 2008 in *Alternative Therapies,* Belinda Wurn and colleagues studied the effects of manual soft tissue techniques to treat blocked fallopian tubes. They studied twenty-eight patients and found that seventeen of them had an improvement in either one or both tubes. This was confirmed either with imaging (hysterosalpingography) or by the fact they managed to have a normal pregnancy.

## Several Types of Pain May Occur
## Due to Different Causes in the Same Person

Ursula Wesselmann has been researching vulvadynia extensively. Vulvadynia is a condition characterized by burning, stinging, irritation, or rawness of the female genital area when there is no apparent infection or skin disease causing these symptoms. She found that several types of pain caused by different pain mechanisms may occur in the same person. For Visceral Manipulation, this reinforces the need for accurate evaluation to discover the particular cause or causes of visceral pain in each person.

## Autonomic Nervous System and Its Relationship
## to Structural Restrictions of the Spine

Charles Henley, Douglas Ivins, Miriam Mills, Frances Wen, and Bruce Benjamin studied seventeen healthy people between the ages of nineteen and fifty to find the effect of neck treatment on vagus nerve tone. This was achieved by measuring the heart rate with an electrocardiograph (ECG) before and after treatment. The reading was compared to times when the subject did not receive treatment, and the findings showed that neck treatment affected the autonomic nervous system and shifted the balance from sympathetic to parasympathetic with treatment. This supports the theories that underpin many of the concepts of Neural Manipulation.

## Emotions and Their Links to Organs

Barral studied the emotional links to organs by observing the behavior and reactions of different patients with specific disorders. Having studied hundreds of patients with a set problem (e.g., hepatitis or colitis) he became aware that they tended to display similar emotional states.

## Case Studies

Many thousands of individual cases have been recorded where Visceral Manipulation seems to have created change. Although they are not organized studies, they are forming a valuable knowledge base that can be utilized for further study and information. Before Jean-Pierre Barral teaches any new technique he has developed, he maintains he has tried it on at least eight hundred patients to check its effectiveness. Through working in hospitals, Barral was fortunate that in cases of more serious pathology he was often able to feel the tissues before a body was either opened up for surgery or scanned. In that way he could test the accuracy of his findings and further refine his techniques.

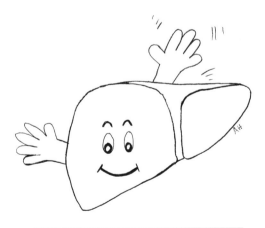

Figure 19.1. After Visceral Manipulation

# Glossary

**Acupuncture**—a branch of traditional medicine developed in China that uses needles to stimulate meridians (energy flow) through the body.

**Acute**—used to describe a condition that develops rapidly or is experienced intensely.

**Adrenal glands**—a pair of glands situated above the kidneys that release hormones to help the body deal with stress.

**Adrenaline** (also Epinephrine, in the U.S.)—a hormone released by the adrenal glands in response to stress and also used at nerve junctions in the body.

**Adson-Wright**—a test done with the patient in a sitting position and involves moving the arm while checking the pulse to test for causes of shoulder, neck, or arm symptoms, or movement restriction.

**Alveolar sacs**—thin membranous bags found in the lungs that allow for gas exchange.

**Alveoli**—part of the lungs consisting of thin membranous sacs that allow for maximum gas exchange.

**Amplitude**—the extent and fullness of a movement.

**Aneurism**—a bulge in a blood vessel that may be caused by disease or weakening of the blood vessel wall and can be dangerous if it gets too large or bursts.

**Anatomy**—the study of the structure of the human body.

**Apnea** (British: Apnoea)—the tendency to stop breathing spontaneously.

**Aorta**—the artery that runs down the midline of the torso and carries blood full of oxygen away from the heart to supply all parts of the body.

**Appendix**—a small finger-like projection from the cecum of the large intestine that has immune functions.

**Arterial system**—the system of the aorta, arteries, and arterioles, which carries oxygenated blood away from the heart toward the rest of the body.

**Arteriole**—the small subdivision of an artery that forms thin-walled vessels ending in capillaries.

**Artery**—a blood vessel carrying oxygenated blood away from the heart toward organs and tissues in the body.

**Autoimmune disease**—condition where an individual produces antibodies that attack their own tissue.

**Autonomic nervous system** (ANS)—the automatic nervous system that controls actions in the body that occur without conscious thought; consists of two parts—the sympathetic and parasympathetic systems.

**Bile**—(also known as gall) a green fluid made by the liver and stored in the gallbladder, which aids the digestion of fats.

**Blood vessels**—tubes, including the aorta, vena cava, arteries, veins, arterioles, venules, and capillaries, which carry blood throughout the body.

**Botox**—the toxin botulinum, which is injected into a nerve junction to stop it from contracting a muscle for a period of about two to three months.

**Bradycardia**—Heartbeat that is slower than the normal expected rate.

**Bronchus** (pleural bronchi)—a tube in the airways that carries air to and from the lungs.

**Cadaver**—a dead body used for medical studies.

**Calcitonin**—a hormone produced by the thyroid gland to regulate calcium balance in the body.

**Capillaries**—the finest blood vessels, which permit the exchange of nutrients and metabolic wastes between the tissues and circulating blood.

**Carbon dioxide**—the gas that is produced as a waste product by the body from oxygen use and then exhaled.

**Carpal tunnel syndrome**—caused by the narrowing of an area in the wrist, leading to pain and weakness in the hand.

**Cecum** (British: *Caecum*)—the first part of the colon, which lies in the lower right abdomen.

**Celiac disease**—an autoimmune disease of the small intestine that indicates that a person is intolerant to gluten.

**Central nervous system**—the brain and spinal cord that form the body's central control system.

**Cerebrospinal Fluid** (CSF)—the fluid that surrounds the brain and spinal cord and is contained within the meninges (bag-like structures around the brain and spinal cord). It is a clear liquid, a little thicker than water, which is extracted from the blood.

**Chiropractor** (practices chiropractic)—a complementary therapist involved in the diagnosis, prevention, and manual correction of mechanical problems in the body, often using manipulation. Chiropractors believe that a structural problem will lead to nervous system dysfunction and symptoms which impact on the health of a person.

**Chronic**—a long-term or slowly developing condition.

**Circulation**—the flow of blood or other fluids within the body.

**Circulatory system**—the system that carries and pumps blood through the body including the blood vessels and heart.

**Clavicle**—the collarbone.

**Cm H2O**—centimeters in water, a measurement of pressure.

**Coarctation of the aorta**—a developmental narrowing of a section of the aorta.

**Coccyx**—the lowest part of the spine, consisting of three to five bone sections that fuse together into a small triangular shaped bone. The tip of the human tail.

**Collagen**—a protein fiber that is strong but not very stretchy; it is one of the components of fascia and muscle.

**Colic**—a condition that usually affects babies, consisting of abdominal pain that starts and stops abruptly, often of undiagnosed causes.

**Colitis**—inflammatory conditions of the large intestine. May have various causes and is often chronic.

**Combined technique**—a VM technique that combines a local hands-on treatment with use of another part of the body as a long lever.

**Complementary healthcare**—various therapies that do not fall into the category of conventional medicine and tend to have belief systems based on helping the body heal itself as naturally as possible (that is without the use of surgery, medication, etc.).

**Congenital**—something existing or dating from birth.

**Conventional Medicine**—mainstream Western medicine as practiced by doctors and nurses, involving use of diagnosis, testing, medication, and surgery.

**Coronary**—of or relating to the heart (e.g., coronary artery is the artery supplying the heart).

**Cortisol**—an adrenal hormone released in response to stress.

**Cranial**—relating to the skull.

**Craniosacral rhythm**—the rhythm created by the change of pressure of the cerebrospinal fluid (CSF) as it is refreshed. It is about twelve to fourteen cycles per minute and is used in CranioSacral therapy to evaluate the state of the body.

**CranioSacral therapy** (CST)—a branch of complementary therapy that is a gentle, hands-on method of evaluating and enhancing the functioning of the membranes and cerebrospinal fluid (CSF) that surround and protect the brain and spinal cord.

**Cyclic**—comes in cycles.

**Cyst**—a sac that is created by the body to wall off an area, usually of infection, fluid, or air.

**Cystic duct**—the tube that carries bile from the gallbladder to the duodenum.

**Diabetes mellitus type 1**—an autoimmune disease of the pancreas that leads to cell dysfunction, causing diabetes.

**Diaphragm**—the large dome-like muscle in the chest that is used for breathing.

**Diastole**—the phase of each heartbeat when the heart relaxes and fills up with blood; the bottom number of a blood pressure reading.

**Differential Listening**—a VM technique of Local Listening over an organ or tissue to find the specific point of restriction.

**Direct Technique** (European definition)—a technique that works directly on a restricted tissue, compressing or stretching it.

**Direct Technique** (US definition)—to work in the direction of direct stretch; stretching a restricted tissue.

**Doppler**—a device that monitors blood flow.

**Duodenum**—the first section of the small intestine, which is about 1 foot (30 cm) long and shaped like an angular "C."

**Dyspepsia**—indigestion.

**Edema** (British: Oedema)—fluid congestion in tissue.

**Elastin**—the stretchy protein fiber that is a component of membranes, skin and fascia.

**Embolism**—piece of the body that is carried through the blood vessels to another part of the body and causes a blockage. This may be a blood clot, fat, or bubble of air, for example.

**Embryological migration**—the way body tissues move during early development in the early stages of pregnancy.

**Endocrine gland**—an organ that produces hormones.

**Endometriosis**—a woman's condition in which the lining of the womb cells are deposited outside the womb.

**Enzymes**—molecules that activate or speed up the rate of chemical reactions.

**Esophagus** (British: *Oesophagus*)—the tube that carries food from the back of the mouth down to the top of the stomach.

**Estrogen** (British: *Oestrogen*)—a female hormone released primarily by the ovaries.

**Expir**—a VM term referring to the passive phase of Motility, in which the organs return along the pathway they followed during early development. Not related to breathing at all.

**Expiration**—breathing out.

**Fallopian Tube**—a tube that runs from the ovary to the uterus to transport the egg.

**Fascia**—a soft tissue membrane in the body that links all parts of the body but also helps keep areas separate from one another. It is smooth and stretchy, and allows easy body movements.

**Fetus** (British: *foetus*)—a developing baby in the womb.

**Fibroid**—a growth in the uterus that is usually benign.

**Fibrous**—made from fibers.

**Fluidity**—having fluid movement.

**Fluoroscopy**—an X-ray imaging technique used to obtain real-time moving images of the internal structures of a patient.

**Fracture**—to break a bone.

**Gallstones**—stones formed from an over-concentration of bile, found in the gallbladder.

**Ganglia** (nerve)—junction point of nerves.

**General Listening**—a VM term for the evaluative technique that gives a practitioner a general idea of where the greatest tension in the body is at that specific time.

**Glenohumeral articulation test**—a test for shoulder Mobility, done with the patient in a seated or lying position as a way of discovering organ restrictions that may be causing shoulder symptoms.

**Goiter** (British: *goitre*)—a swelling of the thyroid gland that can lead to neck swelling.

**Greater omentum**—a membranous apron that hangs from the stomach, folds over and attaches to the transverse colon to form a protective lining of the abdomen.

**Ground substance**—a component of fascia that contains blood vessels, fluid, nutrients, and waste products.

**Hepatic**—relating to the liver.

**Hepatitis**—inflammation of the liver.

**Hiatus hernia**—a protrusion of the upper part of the stomach up through the diaphragm. causing symptoms of heartburn or pain in the chest.

**Holistic**—consideration of all aspects of health, including structural, chemical, emotional, and lifestyle.

**Hormone**—a chemical released by one cell that affects cells in another part of the body.

**HRT** (Hormone Replacement Therapy)—a medication given to women of menopausal age to artificially replace hormones to relieve symptoms of menopause.

**Hyperplasia**—abnormal cell proliferation of cells within an organ or tissue.

**Hypertension**—high blood pressure.

**Hyperthyroidism**—an overactive thyroid, which can lead to symptoms including weight loss, bulging eyes, and hyperactivity.

**Hypothalamus**—part of the brain located just above the brain stem with links to the nerve and hormonal systems.

**Hypothyroidism**—an underactive thyroid, which can lead to symptoms including tiredness and weight gain.

**Ileum**—the final section of the small intestine, composed of 12 feet (4 m) of coiled tubing for the absorption of nutrients.

**Immune System**—the system that protects the body from infection.

**Indirect Technique** (European definition)—working on one tissue to affect another tissue in a different part of the body.

**Indirect Technique** (US definition)—to work in the direction of ease; that is, the direction that has more movement.

**Induction**—a VM technique whereby a tissue is offered encouragement to gain a little extra movement in its direction of ease; that is, the direction that has more movement.

**Inhibition**—a VM technique used to distinguish between several points or areas to find the one that is the primary problem to the body at that time. The practitioner gently supports the area of restriction to stop its affecting the body temporarily.

**Inspir**—a VM term referring to the active phase of Motility where the tissue traces the pathway it followed during early development (nothing to do with breathing).

**Inspiration**—to breathe in.

**Intracranial**—within the skull.

**Intraneural**—within the nerve.

**Intravenous**—within the vein.

**Intrinsic**—within a tissue.

**IUD** (Intrauterine device)—a contraceptive device that is fitted into the uterus.

**IVF** (In vitro fertilization)—a fertility treatment involving fertilizing a women's egg in the laboratory and then putting it into her uterus for pregnancy.

**Jejunoileum**—the jejunum and ileum—in this book referred to as the small intestine.

**Jejunum**—the second section of the small intestine, between the duodenum and the ileum, which is a greatly folded 8-foot-long (2.5 m) tube.

**Jugular foramen**—the opening at the base of the skull through which pass the jugular vein and cranial nerves IX, X, and XI.

**Jugular vein**—the vein that is responsible for eighty percent of the fluid drainage from the head and passes out of the head through the jugular foramen.

**Kinesiology**—a complementary therapy evaluative system involving muscle testing to find problems in the body and help determine preferred treatment options.

**Laparoscopy**—a medical surgical procedure in the abdomen, done using a camera; also known as keyhole surgery.

**Lasègue**—a test used to help determine the cause of sciatica, done with the patient lying on his or her back and involves lifting the leg and monitoring changes in symptoms.

**Lesion**—an osteopathic term for a motion barrier/restriction in the body.

**Listening**—a VM term relating to a physical feeling for evaluation of what is going on in the body.

**Local Listening**—a VM evaluative technique involving a practitioner placing a hand on the body and allowing the hand to be pulled in the direction of the tissue restriction.

**Long lever**—a term used in VM for when a movement of part of the body or active function (such as breathing, swallowing, or moving the leg or arm) is used to help release a restriction.

**Lumbar**—low back area, consisting of five bones in the spine.

**Lymph nodes**—part of the lymphatic system found in various locations in the body; a small capsulated group of cells that filter and trap infections and foreign particles.

**Lymphatic system**—responsible for the circulation and balance of lymph fluid, the fluid balance of cells; has immune functions.

**Manual Thermal Evaluation**—a VM evaluative technique that involves manually scanning the body to detect temperature changes in the tissues as a way to locate restrictions.

**Manipulation**—manual examination and treatment of the body.

**Melatonin**—a hormone that is important in sleep/wake cycles.

**Meninges**—the membranes that cover the central nervous system (brain and spinal cord) including dura, arachnoid, and pia layers.

**Mesentery**—a double layer of membrane that connects an organ to the posterior body wall (spine).

**Metabolism**—the set of automatic chemical reactions that keep humans alive.

**Mobility**—the movement of a tissue in space or against another tissue.

**Mobilization** (British: *Mobilisation*)—movement of a structure or tissue.

**Motility**—the intrinsic active motion of an organ. A rhythmic motion to allow fluids to move through the organ, to allow nutrients to be carried into, and waste products away from, the tissues.

**Musculoskeletal system**—forms the frame of the body; includes the bones, muscles, ligaments, joints, and fascia.

**Myalgic Encephalomyelitis** (ME)—a condition of unknown causes but includes post-infection and leads to debilitating symptoms of widespread muscle and joint pain, cognitive difficulties, chronic, often severe mental and physical exhaustion in a previously healthy and active person. It is called ME reflecting that brain stem swelling is the diagnostic symptom, but is often included under the Chronic Fatigue Syndrome (CFS) umbrella.

**Neural Manipulation** (NM)—a branch of VM that focuses on treatment of the nervous system.

**Neuropathy**—a disorder of the nerves.

**Nervous system**—the control system of the body including brain, spinal cord, and nerves.

**Noradrenalin** (also *Norepinephrine,* in the U.S.)—a hormone and neurotransmitter that influences heart rate and blood flow in response to stress.

**Occiput**—the bone that forms the back and base of the skull.

**Omega-3**—Oils that are essential to the body.

**Omentum** (omenta pleural)—from Latin meaning "apron," it denotes the membrane that joins one organ to another. There is the greater omentum from the stomach to the transverse colon, and the lesser omentum from liver to stomach and duodenum.

**Osteopath** (European definition as is used in this book)—a complementary therapist, who uses a system of diagnosis and treatment that places emphasis on the muscles and bones of the body, often using manipulation and mobilization to restore functioning. In the United States, osteopaths are medical doctors who may or may not use manipulation or work on joints.

**Ovarian**—pertaining to the ovary.

**Ovary** (ies)—a pair of organs found in females in the lower abdomen that make and store eggs.

**Oxygen**—a gas that is essential for life and body functioning; a component of air that the lungs are able to extract and then is carried to the tissues by the blood circulation.

**Oxygenated**—containing oxygen.

**Pancreas**—an organ that crosses the midline of the abdomen; has digestive and endocrine functions.

**Pancreatic duct**—the pipe that links the pancreas to the duodenum through which pancreatic secretions pass into the digestive system.

**Parasympathetic nervous system**—the part of the autonomic nervous system that relaxes the body.

**Parathyrin** (PTH)—a hormone produced by the parathyroid glands.

**Parathyroid glands**—four small glands found in the front of the neck at each corner of the thyroid gland; they release a hormone involved in bone maintenance.

**Pericardium**—the double-layered sac-like structure that surrounds the heart.

**Peripheral**—outside the center.

**Peripheral nervous system**—the network of nerves throughout the body lying outside the central nervous system.

**Peristalsis**—the muscular movements within the digestive system that propel food through the digestive tract.

**Peritoneum** (Peritoneal)—the membrane that lines the abdominal cavity and supports its organs.

**Peyer's patches**—patches on the small intestine that have immune system functions.

**Photon**—the basic unit of light or radiation.

**Physiology**—the study of how the body works.

**Physiotherapist** (Physical therapist)—a therapist, who often works within conventional medicine, who provides services to individuals and populations to develop, maintain, and restore maximum movement and functional ability. They may use manual therapy, rehabilitative therapies, as well as ultrasound and exercises.

**Pineal**—a small gland in the brain that produces hormones especially concerned with sleep/wake cycles.

**Pituitary**—a gland at the base of the brain that produces hormones that regulate many other hormonal glands in the body.

**Pleura**—the double-layered sac-like membranes that encompass each lung.

**Posture/postural analysis**—the study of how a person holds him- or herself in an upright position.

**Prolapse**—literally, "to fall out of place"; used for organs that have become displaced.

**Psoas muscle**—a muscle that runs from the low back spine to the front of the leg and lies behind the kidney. It is responsible for lifting the leg toward the front of the body.

**Psychosomatic illness**—an illness created by the mind but manifesting as physical symptoms.

**Ptosis**—a sagging or prolapse of a tissue.

**Pulse**—the palpable beat of an artery.

**Pyelography**—an X-ray picture of the kidneys, ureters, and bladder.

**Recoil**—a VM technique that involves quickly releasing a compression or tension of a tissue to help energize or "wake up" an area of restriction.

**Reflexes**—automatic, involuntary responses of the body that do not require thought or conscious control.

**Reflexology** (Zone therapy, in some countries)—a complementary therapy most commonly known for working from the feet (but can also be from the hands), which believes that the whole body is reflected on these areas. Using manual techniques, evaluation and treatment is made through assessment, and stimulation of the reflex points on the feet or hands.

**Rehabilitative techniques**—techniques used to restore as normal a function as possible following physical disability.

**Renal**—related to the kidneys.

**Restriction**—an area that is not able to move properly and often will pull surrounding tissue toward it.

**Rolfer**—someone who practices Rolfing, a complementary therapy developed by Ida Rolf that uses soft tissue manipulation and movement education to organize and re-align the whole body in relationship to gravity.

**Sacrum**—a large, triangular bone at the base of the spine and back part of the pelvis; made of five bones that fuse together around the age of sixteen.

**Sciatica**—inflammation of the sciatic nerve, and commonly used to refer to leg pain due to nerve problems.

**Septum**—a partition dividing compartments.

**Seratonin**—a neurotransmitter made in the central nervous system and intestine that has a role in mood and feelings of relaxation and well-being.

**Sheath**—a wrapping.

**Shiatsu**—a complementary therapy developed in Japan that uses massage along meridians (energy lines) in the body.

**Shingles** (herpes zoster)—a virus.

**Sigmoid colon**—the last part of the large intestine, which links the colon to the rectum and lies in the left pelvic area.

**Sjögren's syndrome**—an autoimmune condition.

**Sphenoid**—a bone in the skull located behind the eyes and above the mouth.

**Sphincter of Oddi**—the valve where the cystic and pancreatic ducts enter the duodenum.

**Sphincters**—transition valves that manage the flow of digestion.

**Spleen**—an organ located to the left side under the lower ribs that has immune functions and produces blood cells.

**Sprain**—a joint injury that involves ligament damage.

**Stacking**—a VM technique that involves a practitioner's working in multiple planes of motion to affect the tissue. Done to increase the tension on an area in several dimensions of motion—up and down, left to right, rotationally, and front to back.

**Stenosis**—narrowing usually of a vessel or canal.

**Sternum**—breastbone, found in front of the chest area centrally, and the ribs connect into it.

**Steroids**—a chemical made from fat found in the body; a type of hormone.

**Strain**—a muscle injury usually due to overstretch or overuse.

**Sympathetic nervous system**—the part of the Autonomic nervous system that is activated when the body is stressed.

**Systemic Lupus Erythematosus** (SLE)—an autoimmune condition that can affect any part of the body.

**Systole**—the phase of each heartbeat when the heart contracts, pushing blood out of the heart; the top number of a blood pressure reading.

**Tachycardia**—a faster than normal heart rate.

**Tarsal tunnel syndrome**—a narrowing of a space in the ankle that can cause pain and numbness in the sole of the foot.

**Temporal bone**—the bone on either side of the skull that contains the ear canal and to which the ear connects.

**Tension tests**—VM term for various tests that involve the practitioner placing the body in a particular position or having the patient perform a particular movement, and then measuring a response, such as pain or range of motion, or checking the pulse. Include Adson-Wright, Lasegue, and Glenohumeral Articulation tests.

**Testicle** (plural: *testes*)—a paired male gland that manufactures sperm and hangs outside the body in the scrotum in order to maintain the correct temperature.

**Thoracic Outlet Syndrome**—a group of disorders caused by compression of either blood vessels or nerves to the arm in the chest or neck region leading to symptoms including arm weakness, numbness, tingling and pain.

**Thrombosis**—a blood clot within a blood vessel.

**Thymus**—a gland in the upper chest between and in front of the lungs; has immune functions. It is larger in children and then shrinks with age.

**Thyroid gland**—situated in the front of the neck; releases hormones that have functions in weight control, metabolism, and energy levels.

**Thyroidian**—relating to the thyroid.

**Thyroxin** (T4)—a hormone produced by the thyroid gland.

**Tissue**—a group of cells that form a structure. In this book it refers to any structure in the body.

**Torticollis**—wry neck, a condition in which the head is tilted toward one side due to muscle spasm.

**Toxins**—waste products in the body or foreign particles that either may cause disease or affect the body.

**Trachea**—the main pipe that carries air from the head to the lungs, then feeds into bronchi.

**Trauma**—an injury, whether physical or mental.

**Triiodothronine** (T3)—a hormone produced by the thyroid gland.

**Ultrasound**—a diagnostic imaging or treatment technique using sound waves.

**Urachus**—a ligament that links the bladder to the naval.

**Ureter**—the pipe that joins each kidney to the bladder.

**Urethra**—the canal that carries urine from the bladder to be excreted.

**Uterus**—womb.

**Vascular system**—blood circulation system.

**Vein**—a blood vessel that carries oxygen-depleted blood from the body tissues toward the heart.

**Vena cava**—one of the large veins by which blood is carried back to the heart from the body.

**Venules**—fine veins that feed from the capillaries into the veins.

**Vertebra(e)**—bone(s) in the spine.

**Vesicoureteral reflux**—an abnormal movement of urine from the bladder back to the kidneys.

**Viscera**—the internal organs.

**Visceral Manipulation** (VM)—a hands-on therapy with the specific goal of improving the functioning of the body by addressing its structural imbalances, tensions, and restrictions, and facilitating normal motion of the body, both within and between the tissues.

**Viscerosomatic reflex**—a reflex by which a problem in an organ is reflected out to a muscle or skin sensation, e.g., pain in the arm due to heart problems.

**Whiplash**—an injury to the neck, often caused by a high-speed car accident; leads to pain and stiffness of neck.

# References

Arnold, Kendra L. 2007. Jean-Pierre Barral, Medical Inventor. *Natural Awakening.* September issue.

Barral, Jean-Pierre. 2005. *Manual Thermal Evaluation.* Seattle, WA: Eastland Press.

Barral, Jean-Pierre. 1991. *The Thorax.* Seattle, WA: Eastland Press.

Barral, Jean-Pierre. 2007. *Understanding the Messages of Your Body: How to Interpret Physical and Emotional Signs to Achieve Optimum Health.* Berkeley, CA: North Atlantic Books.

Barral, Jean-Pierre. 1993. *Urogenital Manipulation.* Seattle, WA: Eastland Press.

Barral, Jean-Pierre. Visceral Manipulation DVD. 2002, 2005. Verlag fuer Ganzheitlicke Medizin Dr. Erich Wuehr GmbH & Eastland Press Inc, Seattle, WA. Available at www.barralinstitute.com.

Barral, Jean-Pierre. 2007. *Visceral Manipulation II Revised Edition.* Seattle, WA: Eastland Press.

Barral, Jean-Pierre and Alain Croibier. 2008. *Manual Therapy for the Cranial Nerves.* Philadelphia, PA: Churchill Livingstone Elsevier.

Barral, Jean-Pierre and Alain Croibier. 2007. *Manual Therapy for the Peripheral Nerves.* Philadelphia, PA: Churchill Livingstone Elsevier.

Barral, Jean-Pierre and Alain Croibier. 2000. *Trauma: An Osteopathic Approach.* Seattle, WA: Eastland Press.

Barral, Jean-Pierre and Alain Croibier. 2008. *Visceral Approach to the Vascular System (VVS).* West Palm Beach, FL: The Barral Institute.

Barral, Jean-Pierre, Alain Croibier, and Gail Wetzler. 2005. *Nervous System: Peripheral Nerve Manipulation Lower Limb Study Guide (NS3).* West Palm Beach, FL: The Barral Institute.

Barral, Jean-Pierre, Alain Croibier, and Gail Wetzler. 2005. *Neural Manipulation: Peripheral Nerve Manipulation Upper Body Study Guide (NM2).* West Palm Beach, FL: The Barral Institute.

Barral, Jean-Pierre and Gail Wetzler. 2004. *Visceral Listening Techniques Study Guide* West Palm Beach, FL: UI Publishing.

Barral, Jean-Pierre and Gail Wetzler. 2005. *Visceral Manipulation: Abdomen 1 Study Guide (VM1)*. West Palm Beach, FL: The Barral Institute.

Barral, Jean-Pierre and Gail Wetzler. 2005. *Visceral Manipulation: ViscecroEmotional Relationships Study Guide* (VM6). West Palm Beach, FL: The Barral Institute.

Barral, Jean-Pierre, Alain Croibier, Gail Wetzler, Barbara LeVan, and Christoph Sommer. 2005. *Nervous System: Neuromeningeal Manipulation Study Guide (NS1)*. West Palm Beach, FL: The Barral Institute.

Barral, Jean-Pierre, Gail Wetzler, Dee Ahern, and Lisa Brady Grant. 2005. *Visceral Manipulation: Abdomen 2 Study Guide (VM2)*. West Palm Beach, FL: The Barral Institute.

Barral, Jean-Pierre and Pierre Mercier. 1988. *Visceral Manipulation*. Seattle, WA: Eastland Press.

Binnebosel, Marcel, Uwe Klinge, Raphael Rosch, Karsten Junge, Petra Lynen-Jansen, and Volker Schumpelick. 2008. Morphology, quality, and composition in mature human peritoneal adhesions. *Langenbecks Arch Surgery.* 393:59–66.

Blower, A.L., A. Brooks, G.C. Fenn, A. Hill, M.Y. Pearce, S. Morant, and K.D. Bardhan. 1997. Emergency admissions for upper gastrointestinal disease and their relation to NSAID use. *Alimentary Pharmacology and Therapeutics.* 11:2.

Castellarin, Ioná B. and Margit Jonassa. 2002. Effect of Visceral Osteopathy on the gastrointestinal abnormalities in children with autistic disorders. *Journal of Osteopathic Medicine.* 5:1.

Diamond, Michael and Michael Freeman. 2001. Clinical implications of post surgical adhesions. *Human Reproduction Update.* 76:567–576.

Finet, Georges and Christian Willaime. 2000. *Treating Visceral Dysfunction: An Osteopathic Approach to Understanding and Treating Abdominal Organs.* Portland OR: Stillness Press.

Henley, Charles E., Douglas Ivins, Miriam Mills, Frances K. Wen, and Bruce A. Benjamin. 2008. Osteopathic manipulative treatment and its relationship to Autonomic nervous system activity as demonstrated by heart rate variability: a repeated measures study. *Osteopathic Medicine and Primary Care.* 2:7 doi:10.1186/1750-4732-2-7.

Nemett, Diane R., Barbara A. Fivush, Ranjiv Mathews, Nathalie Camirand, Marlo A. Eldridge, Kathy Finney, and Arlene C. Gerson. 2008. A randomized controlled trial of the effectiveness of osteopathy-based manual physical therapy in treating pediatric dysfunctional voiding. *Journal of Pediatric Urology.* 4:100–106.

Stone, Caroline A. 2006. *Visceral and Obstetric Osteopathy.* Philadelphia, PA: Churchill Livingstone Elsevier.

Upledger Institute. 2005. *Manual Thermal Evaluation and VisceroEmotional 1 Notebook.* West Palm Beach, FL: UI Publishing.

Ward, Robert C. 2007. *Foundations for Osteopathic Medicine,* 2nd edition. London. Lippincott Williams & Wilkins.

Wesselmann, Ursula. 2002. *Vulvodynia Workshop Highlights Prevalence of Disorder: Scientists Share Findings on Pain Research and New Therapies.* National Institute of Health News Release. June 23, 2002. www.nichd.nih.gov/news/releases/vulvodynia.cfm

Wetzler, Gail. 1994. *A Clinical Study on the Effects of Visceral Manipulation for Low Back Spinal Dysfunction.* The Institute of Graduate Physical Therapy and The International Federation of Orthopaedic Manipulative Therapists. Abstracts from the 5th International Conference of the International Federation of Orthopaedic Manipulative Therapists. June 1–5, 1992.

Wetzler, Gail. 2004. *Visceral Manipulation 4: The Thorax Study Guide.* West Palm Beach, FL: UI Publishing.

Wetzler, Gail and Jean-Pierre Barral. 2005. *Visceral Manipulation 3: The Pelvis Study Guide.* West Palm Beach, FL: UI Publishing.

Wurn, Belinda F., Lawrence J. Wurn, C. Richard King, Marvin A. Heuer, Amanda S. Roscow, Kimberley Hornberger, and Eugenia S. Scharf. 2008. Treating fallopian tube occlusion with a manual pelvic physical therapy. *Alternative Therapies.* 141:18–23

Zollars, Jean Anne and Gail Wetzler. 2008. *Visceral Manipulation: Applications for Pediatrics Study Guide (VAP).* West Palm Beach FL: The Barral Institute.

# About the Author

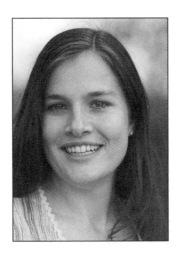

Alison Harvey is a trained practitioner in modalities that include chiropractic, Applied Kinesiology, CranioSacral Therapy, and Visceral Manipulation. After five years of study at the Anglo-European College of Chiropractic in Bournemouth, England, she graduated with a BSc degree in Human Sciences and an MSc degree in chiropractic. She was also awarded the Holm Award for her holistic approach to patient care. She has had extensive training in Visceral Manipulation from the Barral Institute and she oversees the Barral Institute UK (www.barralinstitute.co.uk). She also teaches CranioSacral Therapy internationally for the Upledger Institute. Currently living in Ayr, Scotland, she runs a busy multidisciplinary natural health center. Her treatment approach combines Visceral Manipulation, chiropractic, CranioSacral Therapy, and Applied Kinesiology to give a comprehensive approach to patient care. More information about Alison Harvey and her work can be found online at www.ayrchiropractic.co.uk.

# About North Atlantic Books

North Atlantic Books (NAB) is an independent, nonprofit publisher committed to a bold exploration of the relationships between mind, body, spirit, and nature. Founded in 1974, NAB aims to nurture a holistic view of the arts, sciences, humanities, and healing. To make a donation or to learn more about our books, authors, events, and newsletter, please visit www.northatlanticbooks.com.

North Atlantic Books is the publishing arm of the Society for the Study of Native Arts and Sciences, a 501(c)(3) nonprofit educational organization that promotes cross-cultural perspectives linking scientific, social, and artistic fields. To learn how you can support us, please visit our website.